PCR PROTOCOLS
in
MOLECULAR TOXICOLOGY

CRC Press
METHODS IN TOXICOLOGY

Edward J. Massaro - *Advisory Editor*
Senior Research Scientist
National Health and Environmental Effects Research Laboratory
Research Triangle Park, North Carolina

The **CRC Press Methods in Toxicology Series** provides the reader with a step-by-step approach to each of the up-to-date methods and techniques presented in a clear and concise format. Topics covering all aspects of the methods that impact on toxicology are being reviewed for publication.

Published Titles

Methods in Renal Toxicology, Rudolfs K. Zalups and Lawrence H. Lash
Molecular and Cellular Methods in Developmental Toxicology, George P. Daston
PCR Protocols in Molecular Toxicology, John P. Vanden Heuvel
Methods in Inhalation Toxicology, Robert F. Phalen

CRC Press
METHODS IN THE LIFE SCIENCES

Gerald D. Fasman - *Advisory Editor*
Brandeis University

Series Overview

Methods in Biochemistry
John Hershey
Department of Biological Chemistry
University of California

Cellular and Molecular Neuropharmacology
Joan M. Lakoski
Department of Pharmacology
Penn State University

Research Methods for Inbred Laboratory Mice
John P. Sundberg
The Jackson Laboratory
Bar Harbor, Maine

Methods in Neuroscience
Sidney A. Simon
Department of Neurobiology
Duke University

Joseph M. Corless
Department of Cell Biology,
Neurobiology and Ophthalmology
Duke University

Methods in Pharmacology
John H. McNeill
Professor and Dean
Faculty of Pharmaceutical Science
The University of British Columbia

Methods in Signal Transduction
Joseph Eichberg, Jr.
Department of Biochemical and Biophysical Sciences
University of Houston

Methods in Toxicology
Edward J. Massaro
Senior Research Scientist
National Health and Environmental Effects Research Laboratory
Research Triangle Park, North Carolina

PCR PROTOCOLS *in* MOLECULAR TOXICOLOGY

Edited by
John P. Vanden Heuvel
Department of Veterinary Science
Penn State University
State College, Pennsylvania

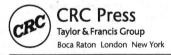

CRC Press is an imprint of the
Taylor & Francis Group, an **informa** business

CRC Press
Taylor & Francis Group
6000 Broken Sound Parkway NW, Suite 300
Boca Raton, FL 33487-2742

© 1998 by Taylor & Francis Group, LLC
CRC Press is an imprint of Taylor & Francis Group, an Informa business

No claim to original U.S. Government works

ISBN-13: 978-0-8493-3344-6 (pbk)
ISBN-13: 978-1-138-47369-0 (hbk)

This book contains information obtained from authentic and highly regarded sources. Reasonable efforts have been made to publish reliable data and information, but the author and publisher cannot assume responsibility for the validity of all materials or the consequences of their use. The authors and publishers have attempted to trace the copyright holders of all material reproduced in this publication and apologize to copyright holders if permission to publish in this form has not been obtained. If any copyright material has not been acknowledged please write and let us know so we may rectify in any future reprint.

Except as permitted under U.S. Copyright Law, no part of this book may be reprinted, reproduced, transmitted, or utilized in any form by any electronic, mechanical, or other means, now known or hereafter invented, including photocopying, microfilming, and recording, or in any information storage or retrieval system, without written permission from the publishers.

For permission to photocopy or use material electronically from this work, please access www. copyright.com (http://www.copyright.com/) or contact the Copyright Clearance Center, Inc. (CCC), 222 Rosewood Drive, Danvers, MA 01923, 978-750-8400. CCC is a not-for-profit organization that provides licenses and registration for a variety of users. For organizations that have been granted a photocopy license by the CCC, a separate system of payment has been arranged.

Trademark Notice: Product or corporate names may be trademarks or registered trademarks, and are used only for identification and explanation without intent to infringe.

Visit the Taylor & Francis Web site at
http://www.taylorandfrancis.com

and the CRC Press Web site at
http://www.crcpress.com

Library of Congress Cataloging-in-Publication Data

PCR protocols in molecular toxicology / edited by John P. Vanden
   Heuvel.
       p. cm. — (CRC Press methods in toxicology)
   Includes bibliographical references and index.
   ISBN 0-8493-3344-X (alk. paper)
    1. Molecular toxicology—Laboratory manuals. 2. Polymerase chain
reaction—Laboratory manuals. I. Vanden Heuvel, John P.
  II. Series.
  RA1220.3.P37 1997
  615.9—dc21   97-20678
                                                CIP

Library of Congress Card Number 97-20678

Editor

John P. Vanden Heuvel, Ph.D., is currently an assistant professor in the Department of Veterinary Science at the Pennsylvania State University, University Park. Dr. Vanden Heuvel is a faculty member of the Molecular Toxicology Program within the Life Science Consortium and the Environmental Resources Research Institute as well as the Pathobiology Program of the Department of Veterinary Science. Dr. Vanden Heuvel received his B.S. degree in pharmacology and toxicology, and his Ph.D. in 1991 in environmental toxicology from the University of Wisconsin–Madison. Subsequently, he received postdoctoral training at the National Institute of Environmental Health Sciences in Research Triangle Park, NC, in the Laboratory of Biochemical Risk Analysis. Prior to accepting his present position at Penn State University, Dr. Vanden Heuvel was an assistant professor of pharmacology and toxicology at Purdue University in West Lafayette, IN.

Dr. Vanden Heuvel is a member of the Society of Toxicology, the American Association of Cancer Research, and the American Association for the Advancement of Science. He has published and presented research in a variety of national and international journals of toxicology, biochemistry, and molecular biology. He also teaches courses in molecular toxicology, molecular carcinogenesis, and pharmacology. Dr. Vanden Heuvel has received research grants from the National Institutes of Health (National Institute of Diabetes and Digestive and Kidney Disorders, National Institute of Environmental Health Sciences), Zeneca Pharmaceutical, Searle-Monsanto, National Toxicology Program, American Institute of Cancer Research, National Cattlemen's Beef Association, and a variety of university- and state-sponsored programs. He is currently researching the signal transduction pathways utilized by fatty acid-like tumor-promoting chemicals as well as endogenous lipids in mammalian cells.

Contributors

John P. Vanden Heuvel, Ph.D.
Department of Veterinary Science
Penn State University
University Park, Pennsylvania

William B. Mattes, Ph.D.
Genetic Toxicology Group
Pharmacia and Upjohn
Kalamazoo, Michigan

J. Christopher Corton, Ph.D.
Chemical Industry Institute of Toxicology
Research Triangle Park, North Carolina

Douglas A. Bell, Ph.D.
Laboratory of Computational Biology and Risk Management
National Institute of Environmental Health Sciences
Research Triangle Park, North Carolina

Gary Pittman
University of North Carolina
Chapel Hill, North Carolina

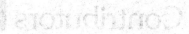

Table of Contents

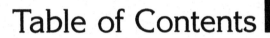

Chapter 1. The Basics of the Polymerase Chain Reaction 1
William B. Mattes

Chapter 2. Analysis of Gene Expression 41
John P. Vanden Heuvel

Chapter 3. Differential Display PCR 99
J. Christopher Corton

Chapter 4. Cloning by PCR 121
John P. Vanden Heuvel

Chapter 5. Genotype Analysis 163
Douglas A. Bell and Gary Pittman

Chapter 6. General Molecular Biology Techniques 177
John P. Vanden Heuvel

Appendix I — List of Suppliers 213

Appendix II — Companies, Online Catalogs, and Internet Resources 217

Index 219

Preface

This book was conceived as a result of a continuing education course, "PCR Applications in Molecular Toxicology," that was taught at the 1996 Society of Toxicology meeting in Anaheim, California. The response from the meeting formed the impetus for the design of this book, as many people expressed a desire to learn more about the technical aspects of the polymerase chain reaction. In addition, since molecular toxicology is an emerging discipline with a diverse set of scientific problems to be addressed, many participants in the course were interested in how to fully utilize the powerful techniques of PCR.

The course not only identified a need in the constituency of the Society of Toxicology but also revealed a gap in most manuals that deal with the polymerase chain reaction. In this book, we have tried to go into more detail about the theory of PCR as well as provide detailed instructions on how to adapt the procedure to various issues of toxicologic interest. We will discuss the basic components of PCR and steps required for optimizing the lab space and the reagents involved. In subsequent chapters specific techniques are discussed in detail, including: quantitative reverse transcriptase PCR and methods to examine gene expression; differential display cloning, a powerful technique to clone toxicant-inducible genes; cloning and library screening by PCR; and genotype and polymorphism analysis of drug and toxicant metabolizing enzymes. Finally, a review of basic, nonPCR-based molecular biology methods that are useful in performing the protocols in prior chapters is discussed.

For the reader's information: Chapter 1 was submitted by William Mattes; Chapters 2, 4, and 6 were written by John Vanden Heuvel; Chapter 3 was submitted by Chris Corton, and; Chapter 5 was written by Douglas Bell and Gary Pittman. John Vanden Heuvel attempted to provide consistency to the overall effort. All the authors hope that you find this handbook useful and that you appreciate the power and complexity of the polymerase chain reaction and can utilize the techniques discussed to advance the field of molecular toxicology. We also hope that the general scientific community will find these approaches useful in their molecular biology research efforts.

D. Bell
C. Corton
W. Mattes
G. Pittman
J. Vanden Heuvel
April 1997

Chapter 1

The Basics of the Polymerase Chain Reaction

William Mattes

Contents

I.	Theory and History of PCR	2
	A. Beginnings	2
	B. Basic Mathematical Considerations	3
	C. Plateau and Limits of Detection	5
II.	The PCR Laboratory	6
	A. Layout and Contamination Control	6
	B. Handling PCR Reagents	8
	C. Working with Small Volumes and Tubes	9
III.	Obtaining a Nucleic Acid Sequence	9
	A. Access to GenBank™ through Email	10
	B. Access to GenBank through the World Wide Web	16
IV.	Primer Design	21
	A. Primer Characteristics	21
	B. Primer Design Using OLIGO® Software	23
	C. Primer Design Using PRIMER	26
	D. Primer Design Using PRIMER 3.0, World Wide Web Version	28
	E. Primer Synthesis	28
V.	PCR Procedure and Optimization	28
	A. Basic Considerations	28
	B. Basic Protocol for Oil-Overlay Thermocyclers	30

0-8493-3344-X/98/$0.00+$.50
© 1998 by CRC Press LLC

C.	DNA Sample for Optimization	31
D.	Optimization Experiment 1 — Cycle Number	31
E.	Optimization Experiment 2 — Annealing Temperature	32
F.	Optimization Experiment 3 — Hot Start	33
G.	Optimization Experiment 4 — MgCl$_2$ Concentration	35
H.	Additives and Other Optimization Approaches	37

Materials Needed ... 37
References ... 38

I. Theory and History of PCR

A. Beginnings

Often the simplest concepts elude the scientific world until they burst upon one individual in a moment of insight. Thus it was on a Friday night, an oligonucleotide chemist, on his way to a weekend in the California mountains and struggling with the technical problems of his experiments, came upon a concept that has indeed revolutionized molecular biology. Perhaps if the road had not been so quiet the scientific world might have had to wait even longer for this unique tool. Fortunately, Kary Mullis was not distracted, and that night he envisioned a process that (like the chain reaction in nuclear fission) gives rise to two products after each reaction cycle, each being a substrate in the next cycle. The process was dependent upon DNA polymerase, and hence was dubbed the polymerase chain reaction (PCR).[1] Over the past decade use of PCR has grown exponentially because of its high sensitivity, simplicity, and flexibility.

The first letter in the acronym PCR stands for DNA polymerase. The characteristics of this enzyme make PCR possible. All known DNA polymerases require deoxyribonucleotide triphosphates (dNTPs), a divalent cation (Mg^{2+} or Mn^{2+}), a DNA template, and a region of that template that is double-stranded adjacent to a single-stranded nick or gap (or continuous single-stranded template) (see Figure 1.1). The double-stranded region (i.e., the primer) must terminate with a 3'-end available for subsequent nucleotide addition. The requirement for a primer region sets the stage for PCR.

DNA synthesis, on a theoretical basis, will continue from the priming region to the end of the template strand. Consider a primer region consisting of a short oligonucleotide hydrogen bonded (i.e., hybridized) to the complementary sequence of a much longer single-stranded polynucleotide. DNA polymerase adds nucleotides to the 3'-end of the oligonucleotide, making a *copy* of the polynucleotide, until it falls off the end of the polynucleotide. The result is a double-stranded DNA molecule. If the double-stranded DNA molecule is denatured (i.e., the two strands are separated) by heat, for example, and once again an oligonucleotide is hybridized to the template, the

The Basics of the Polymerase Chain Reaction

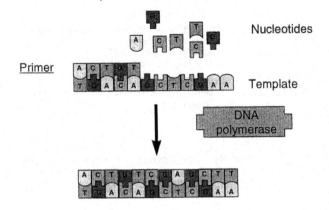

Figure 1.1
Requirement for a DNA primer in DNA synthesis.

process will be repeated. In every cycle, another copy of the complementary strand will be produced, its 5'-end determined by the position of the hybridized oligonucleotide.

Kary Mullis realized that if the starting mixture includes not only a single-stranded polynucleotide template, but also (1) its complementary strand, and (2) two oligonucleotide primers that hybridize to both strands, copies of *both* of these strands will be produced each cycle. These copies can be used as templates for subsequent cycles. Furthermore, short strands whose 5'- and 3'-ends are defined by the position of the two oligonucleotide primers, will accumulate in exponential fashion, i.e., like a chain reaction (Figure 1.2).

B. Basic Mathematical Considerations

As it is commonly carried out the PCR is a rather simple reaction mixture. The components of the control reaction supplied in Perkin Elmer's basic kit

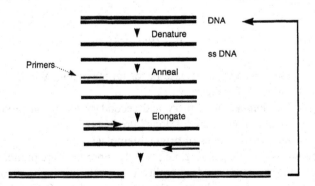

Figure 1.2
Basic PCR diagram.

TABLE 1.1
Lambda Control PCR — From Perkin Elmer

200 μM (each) dNTP   total [dNTPs] = 0.8 mM
Total [MgCl₂ = 1.5 mM   Free [MgCl₂] = 0.7 mM
Bacteriophage Lambda DNA template   Number of cycles = 25
2.5 Units *Taq* DNA Pol per 100 μL   Buffer: 10 mM Tris-HCl, pH 8.3 (at 25°C);
    50 mM KCl

	Before PCR			After PCR		
	Weight	Molarity	Molecules	Weight	Molarity	Molecules
Template (48,500 bp)	1 ng	3.10 e–13	1.86 e7	1 ng	3.00 e–13	1.81 e7
Target (500 bp)	10 pg	3.00 e–13	1.81 e7	1 μg	3.00 e–8	1.81 e12
Primers (25-mers)	1623 ng	2.00 e–6	1.20 e14	1574 ng	1.94 e–6	1.17 e14
dNTPs	39 μg	8.00 e–4	4.82 e16	37 μg	7.70 e–4	4.64 e16
Magnesium Ion	3.6 μg	1.50 e–3	9.03 e16	3.6 μg	1.50 e–3	9.03 e16
Taq DNA polymerase	12.5 ng	1.33 e–9	8.01 e10	12.5 ng	1.33 e–9	8.01 e10

Assumptions and Data:
Taq DNA polymerase specific activity = 250,000 Units/mg
Average MW of a dNTP is 487 Daltons   Average MW of a dNMP is 325 Daltons
Achieve at least 10^5-fold amplification   *Taq* DNA polymerase half-life is not considered

---

are given in Table 1.1, along with their concentrations. The PCR in its simplest form is a combination of a DNA sample, oligonucleotide primers, dNTPs, a thermostable DNA polymerase, and a suitable buffer, heated and cooled repeatedly until a desired amount of "short" DNA product accumulates.

The "short" PCR product is ultimately the product measured. Careful inspection of the product (P) shows that it accumulates according to the formula:

$$P = (Y^n - Yn) \cdot x$$

where Y = the exponential increase factor (at maximum, $Y = 2$)
    n = number of cycles
    Yn = the number of primary and secondary extension products with indeterminate length ("long" products)
    x = number of copies of original template.

Theoretically Y is equal to 2, i.e., two short products are produced during each cycle. On the other hand, in reality Y is rarely this high, often being as low as 1.6 in the author's hands. The efficiency of the PCR refers to how closely this number approaches 2; the efficiency of a reaction with $Y = 1.6$ is

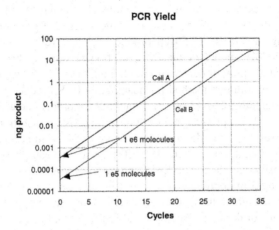

Figure 1.3
Plateau.

60% (i.e., if Y = 1, no amplification has occurred). An important goal of PCR optimization is to increase the efficiency in order to achieve the desired level of amplification with the minimum number of cycles.

C. Plateau and Limits of Detection

Just as a nuclear fission reaction does not continue indefinitely, a PCR eventually reaches a point with increasing cycles where short product fails to accumulate in an exponential fashion. Rather, short product accumulates in a more linear fashion until it stops completely (Figure 1.3). This point is referred to as the plateau. The plateau probably occurs because of a variety of factors. Foremost of these is the eventually overwhelming excess of template over DNA polymerase. For example, Table 1.1 shows the control reaction supplied by Perkin Elmer. Whereas the initial molar ratio of DNA polymerase to template is over 2000:1, it is less than 1:20 when maximum amplification has been achieved. Addition of more *Taq* polymerase to the reaction can increase the maximum yield to an extent,[2] but other factors will still limit the reaction.[3]

The most serious implication of the plateau effect is that when PCR product accumulation changes from an exponential to a linear process, quantitative differences between reaction mixtures cannot be evaluated (Figure 1.3). On the other hand, in the exponential phase (above ~10 cycles) the logarithm of the amount of product is dependent upon the number of cycles, the amount of initial template, and the efficiency of the PCR, i.e., $\log([\text{product}]) = n \cdot \log(Y) + \log(x)$. Thus, a plot of the logarithm of the amount of product as a function of the number of cycles should yield a straight line with slope $\log(Y)$ and intercept $\log(x)$, allowing determination of both Y and initial template concentration in the reaction mixture.[4,5] However, if the PCR begins to enter the plateau phase when the number of molecules of short product equals the number of molecules of *Taq* polymerase, the amount of product will be only about 30 ng (assuming a 350 bp product and 8×10^{10} molecules *Taq* per reaction). A 20% aliquot of the PCR reaction mixture analyzed by electrophoresis is at the limit of detection for ethidium bromide fluorescence (~5 ng). Thus, the most common method for quantitating PCR product is unsuitable at certain cycle numbers. More sensitive methods for product detection (e.g., ^{32}P) can be used to detect product in the exponential phase. In addition, approaches using competitor targets (described elsewhere in this volume) allow quantitation even of plateau phase PCR. The effect of the plateau phase on the PCR must be considered when developing and evaluating a PCR experiment.

A paradigm in approaching the PCR is one that primarily considers the *number of molecules* in the reaction. Dr. Mullis suggests that the concentrations of components of the PCR reaction should be described in terms of *molecules per microliter* rather than molarity or µg per µl.[6] Thus a PCR with 1 ng of lambda DNA in 100 1 (3.1×10^{-13} *M*) contains 1.8×10^7 molecules per µl, i.e., 1.8 u7. Indeed, consideration of numbers of molecules is particularly critical if one is comparing genomic DNA as PCR input with a defined plasmid or PCR product as input. For example, a PCR with a template from 10^5 cells should be compared with a PCR containing 10^5 copies of a control template.

II. The PCR Laboratory

A. Layout and Contamination Control

PCR should not be regarded as just another biochemistry or molecular biology technique. The design of a PCR laboratory should be similar to that in which experiments with viral pathogens or volatile, high-risk radioisotopes are carried out. The primary reason for this is that the end result of a successful PCR is a threat to the success of any subsequent PCR experiments. For example, a PCR starting with 10^4 to 10^5 molecules of target DNA may produce 0.5 µg of DNA product, or 1.4×10^{12} molecules. If the reaction mixture is in a volume of 50 µl, a microscopic drop (e.g., 0.1 µl) would contain 2.8×10^9 molecules! Contamination of a starting reaction with such a droplet ruins that experiment. Contamination of stock reagents used to prepare starting reactions will have a devastating effect on the entire project. Some workers have proposed that "PCR contamination be considered as a form of infection."[7] The healthiest approach is to treat reactions after PCR as if they were highly radioactive or as if they contained a high titer of a very stable pathogenic virus. Other sources of contamination are possible, particularly plasmid or probe preparations containing target sequences, but the primary focus for contamination should always be the solutions and material encountered after PCR. This perspective

The Basics of the Polymerase Chain Reaction

on the potential for contamination in the laboratory should be central to the design and layout of a PCR laboratory.

As a first step in preventing contamination, there should be **strict separation between pre-PCR and post-PCR operations**. All preparations for PCR should be done in one area, but the PCR process and subsequent manipulations and analysis of the reaction mixture should be carried out in a separate area, preferably a different room. If this is not possible, a separate enclosure for either pre-PCR or post-PCR operations, or an enclosure for each operation, should be considered. Enclosures designed for PCR with built-in ultraviolet sterilization are available (e.g., from Oncor, USA Scientific, Inc., Coy Laboratory Products, Inc.), but enclosures designed for radioisotope work (e.g., Scotlab) may suffice. Finally, laminar flow hoods are excellent options for isolating one or both of these operations.

Separation between pre-PCR and post-PCR applies not just to operations, but to all reagents and equipment. Obviously cost and practicality do enter into consideration, however, two sets of the following items should be maintained:

- Tubes
- Pipette tips
- Gloves
- Racks
- Tube openers
- Ice buckets
- Pipettors
- Microcentrifuges
- Reagents

These items should be conspicuously labeled as either PRE-PCR or POST-PCR. Any time equipment from one area is to be used in another it should be thoroughly decontaminated. Separate lab coats for the different areas might also be considered. Some investigators have proposed even more extensive separation, including separate areas for sample preparation, pre-PCR setup, and post-PCR work, with different personnel carrying out different operations, and different operations being carried out on different days.[7] A sense of how and where contamination is generated is the key to setting up the successful PCR laboratory.

As another precaution, all stock reagents used for setting up PCR reaction mixtures should be aliquoted, and the aliquot currently in use identified. Thus, if contamination is suspected, the aliquots of stocks currently in use may be discarded and replaced. As noted above, reagents for pre-PCR and post-PCR work (e.g., EDTA solutions, buffers, etc.) should be segregated.

Care should be taken in all procedures. Sample handling should be minimized, and tubes opened very carefully (preferably with a tube opener that can be easily decontaminated). Gloves should be changed frequently. Aerosol-filtered pipette tips or positive displacement pipettors should always be used. Tips should never be touched by anything but the pipettor (no hands!) nor be put back into the box. The filtered tips are sterile upon arrival, and it is best

8 PCR Protocols in Molecular Toxicology

to keep the top on the box when they are not in use. All plasticware and glassware used in preparing PCR reactions should be purchased sterile or autoclave sterilized (although this will not eliminate DNA contamination, as noted below). The contents of an unopened bag of plasticware (e.g., micro-centrifuge tubes or reaction tubes) may be considered quite free of contamination. **Never remove plasticware from a stock bag with bare hands.** Use gloves, or preferably simply pour the plasticware out of the bag to prevent contamination of the rest of its contents. Similarly, unused plasticware should not be returned to a stock bag.

Finally, in setting up the PCR laboratory, one should consider approaches for decontaminating surfaces, equipment, and possibly solutions. Alcohol and autoclave treatments are ineffective. One of the earliest decontamination methods was sterilization with ultraviolet light.[8] Another method calls for replacing dTTP in the reaction mixture with dUTP. Treatment of pre-PCR mixtures with uracil deoxyribose N-glycosylase (UNG) degrades any contaminating PCR product (i.e., oligonucleotides containing deoxyuridine residues).[9] A simple decontamination method is to treat surfaces and equipment with 10% Clorox®.[10] This treatment is particularly effective for fragile glassware such as quartz cuvettes. By contrast, Pyrex® glassware may be decontaminated by dry-heat baking at 350°F for 3 to 4 hours.

B. Handling PCR Reagents

PCR reagents should be handled carefully to prevent degradation. The most sensitive reagents are the enzymes, e.g., reverse transcriptase, RNase inhibitor, and DNA polymerases. Gloves should be worn at all times when handling these and other PCR reagents to prevent minute flakes of dead skin (which contain proteases and nucleases) from getting into reagents. Proteases and nucleases can digest and inactivate PCR enzymes and nucleic acids, so gloves are a simple precaution.

Enzymes are almost always stored as solutions in glycerol at –20°C, hence they never really freeze. **Enzymes can be "killed" by warming them and then cooling them.** To protect them from the freeze–thaw cycles that all frost-free freezers go through, enzymes should be stored in special boxes containing coolant (from Nalgene or Stratagene), hence preventing changes in temperature. When using enzymes at the lab bench, keep the enzymes in the coolant boxes at all times. The enzyme should not be kept out of the freezer for extended periods.

Finally, other reagents, including buffers, dNTPs, oligonucleotides, RNA, or DNA, may be stored as frozen solutions and need to be thawed. Buffers may be warmed and left at room temperature, but once the dNTPs and oligonucleotide solutions have thawed, they should be vortexed and stored on ice to prevent degradation. RNA should be stored at –120° F and preferably thawed

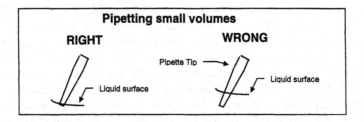

Figure 1.4
Correct small volume pipetting.

on ice; certainly as soon as the solution is melted it should be kept on ice. All solutions should be mixed well before using.

C. Working with Small Volumes and Tubes

The total volume of PCR mixtures is usually between 10 and 100 µl. Thus additions are very small, sometimes less than 1 µl (requiring a pipettor accurate in this range and appropriate tips). If the pipette tip is submerged into the sample, quite a bit of sample will coat the outside of the tip, and the volume delivered to the reaction will be larger than intended. Instead, the pipette tip should be touched to the surface of the sample (Figure 1.4). Obviously, another source of error in such operations is the pipettor itself. To ensure reproducibility, **pipettors should be calibrated on a regular basis**, at least every six months.

III. Obtaining a Nucleic Acid Sequence

Since the key to PCR is a pair of oligonucleotide primers of defined sequence, any PCR experiment begins with DNA sequence information. Usually this DNA sequence is the target of interest but, if those data are unknown, it may be the sequence of a related gene. Thus, the first step of PCR is to gather information. While this may involve a library search, the preferred method is the automated computer search of DNA sequence databases and retrieval of the DNA sequence as a computer file to be used in subsequent primer design. Indeed, the computer is as necessary an element in the PCR laboratory as the pipettor and thermal cycler, and literacy with electronic mail, World Wide Web (Internet) browsing, computer-file formats, and different software packages is essential in developing a PCR research program.

As noted above, the first step in designing PCR primers is obtaining a DNA sequence, and the most convenient way to do so is from GenBank™, the database of all known nucleotide and protein sequences, maintained at the

10 PCR Protocols in Molecular Toxicology

National Center for Biotechnology Information (NCBI) branch of the NIH. GenBank is part of the International Nucleotide Sequence Database Collaboration, which includes the DNA DataBank of Japan (DDBJ) and the European Molecular Biology Laboratory (EMBL). Entries in the database contain, in addition to the sequence data, a description of the sequence, the source organism, complete bibliographic references, and a table of features that identifies coding regions and other sites of biological significance. The information is primarily obtained by direct submission from authors, secondarily by scanning the journal literature, and there is no systematic approach to assuring standard nomenclature. Thus as one searches for DNA sequences for the rat Cyp2B1 gene, one should also consider older nomenclature, such as P450e (see reference 11). GenBank can be searched, and entries retrieved, over the Internet by either direct access to its World Wide Web site through a browser such as Netscape, or indirectly through Internet electronic mail (Email). Both methods will be discussed.

A.   Access to GenBank™ through Email

Electronic mail access to GenBank is through a mail server in which the electronic mail is received by a computer program that analyzes and processes the commands found in the message. The GenBank mail server address is retrieve@ncbi.nlm.nih.gov and a comprehensive set of instructions can be obtained by sending a message like the following:

```
From: your.address@your.institution

Date: 2 Jan 1997 21:29:02-EDT

To: retrieve@ncbi.nlm.nih.gov

Subject:

HELP
```

In minutes a text file will be returned that can be printed and referred to at a later time. For the purposes of example a search will be conducted for sequences for the mouse thymidine kinase gene. The message to send looks like this:

The Basics of the Polymerase Chain Reaction

From: your.address@your.institution

Date: 2 Jan 1997 21:29:02-EDT

To: retrieve@ncbi.nlm.nih.gov

Subject: TK search

DATALIB genbank

MAXDOCS 300

MAXLINES 2000

TITLES

BEGIN

"thymidine kinase" AND mouse

As described in the HELP text received from GenBank, the first line of the message (DATALIB genbank) instructs GenBank to search both the main database and any updates. MAXDOCS 300 tells GenBank to send no more than 300 entries; MAXLINES 2000 limits any one entry to 2000 lines, and TITLES restricts the output to just titles, no sequences. The rationale for this approach is obvious once the return message is examined. Finally, BEGIN tells GenBank that the search criteria are following.

The actual search uses Boolean logic and operators, and one can group searches. By enclosing "thymidine kinase" in quotes the entire phrase is searched for, rather than each word by itself (i.e., thymidine kinase without quotes would pick up thymidine or kinase by itself).

The message that is returned looks like this:

Date: 24-Nov-96 17:30 EST

From: RETRIEVE E-Mail Server > your.address@your.institution

Subj: Results-RETRIEVE Server:tk

===

To Obtain Help Documentation: send e-mail to 'retrieve@ncbi.nlm.nih.gov'
with the word 'help' in the body of the mail message.

Note: GenBank retrieval and submission tools are available through
the World Wide Web at the URL: http://www.ncbi.nlm.nih.gov/ For more
information contact User Services at: info@ncbi.nlm.nih.gov

===

Database: GenBank Updates (97.0+, 11/24/96)

Query: "thymidine kinase" AND mouse

Parse status: OK: 2 documents retrieved.

Documents selected: 1-2 (up to 2000 lines)

1) [AA103707] mo40f03.r1 Life Tech mouse embryo 15 5dpc 10667012 Mus musculus
   cDNA clone 556061 5' similar to gb:K02581 THYMIDINE KINASE,
   CYTOSOLIC (HUMAN); gb:M68489 Mouse thymidine kinase gene, complete
   cds (MOUSE);.

2) [AA110621] mm89b03.r1 Stratagene mouse embryonic carcinoma RA (#937318) Mus
   musculus cDNA clone 535565 5' similar to gb:M68489 Mouse thymidine
   kinase gene, complete cds (MOUSE);.

Database: GenBank (97.0, 10/21/96)

Query: "thymidine kinase" AND mouse

Parse status: OK: 40 documents retrieved.

Documents selected: 1-40 (up to 2000 lines)

1) [MUSTKM] Mouse thymidine kinase gene, complete cds.

2) [MUSTK5F] Mouse thymidine kinase gene, exons 1 and 2 (partial).

3) [SYNMUSHSV] Artificial gene (reporter) constructed of mouse major urinary
   protein (Mup) gene, promoter region and herpes simple virus type 1
   thymidine kinase (HSV tk) gene, partial cds.
4) [MMTKP] Mouse thymidine kinase gene promoter.

5) [SYNMETITK] mouse mt-i gene promoter fused to herpes virus tk gene.

6) [AA000260] mg32b11.r1 Soares mouse embryo NbME13.5 14.5 Mus musculus cDNA
   clone 425469 5' similar to gb:K02581 THYMIDINE KINASE, CYTOSOLIC
   (HUMAN); gb:M68489 Mouse thymidine kinase gene, complete cds
   (MOUSE);.

The Basics of the Polymerase Chain Reaction

11) [W96937] mf60h08.r1 Soares mouse embryo NbME13.5 14.5 Mus musculus cDNA clone 418719 5′ similar to gb:K02581 THYMIDINE KINASE, CYTOSOLIC (HUMAN); gb:M68489 Mouse thymidine kinase gene, complete cds (MOUSE);.

12) [MMTKEX12] M.musculus thymidine kinase gene (exon 1 & 2).

13) [MMTKP1] Murine thymidine kinase processed pseudogene.

14) [MUSTKAA] Mouse cytosolic thymidine kinase mRNA clone pMtk4, complete cds.

15) [MUSTKB] Mouse cytosolic thymidine kinase mRNA clone pMtk9, complete cds.

16) [AA033141] mi39d04.r1 Soares mouse embryo NbME13.5 14.5 Mus musculus cDNA clone 465895 5′ similar to gb:M68489 Mouse thymidine kinase gene, complete cds (MOUSE);.

29) [W90878] mf74c10.r1 Soares mouse embryo NbME13.5 14.5 Mus musculus cDNA clone 420018 5′ similar to gb:M68489 Mouse thymidine kinase gene, complete cds (MOUSE);.

30) [ASU18466] African swine fever virus, complete genome.

31) [MUSTCREC1] Mouse (transgenic MyK-103) segment 1 of integrated DNA.

32) [S57244] tk-1 (tkb+)=thymidine kinase [mice, L5178Y 3.7.2C lymphoma cells, mRNA, 779 nt].

33) [MMREP4] Mouse rearranged major satellite repeat flanking tk insertion site from LC2 cells with microinjected pBR322 containing herpes thymidine kinase (tk) gene.

34) [SYNPBRMU1] HSV tk/pBR322 recombination junction in plasmid rescued from mouse L cells (transformant cell line 1-2-75) transfected with pBR322 and Herpes simplex virus thymidine kinase (HSV tk) gene DNA.

37) [SYNPBRMUA] PBR322/pBR322 recombination junction in plasmid rescued from mouse L cells (transformant cell line 1-2-75) transfected with pBR322 and Herpes simplex virus thymidine kinase (HSV tk) gene DNA.

38) [SYNPBRMUB] PBR322/HSV tk recombination junction in plasmid rescued from mouse L cells (transformant cell line 1-2-75) transfected with pBR322 and Herpes simplex virus thymidine kinase (HSV tk) gene DNA.

39) [SYNPBRMUC] PBR322/pBR322 recombination junction in plasmid rescued from mouse L cells (transformant cell line 1-2-75) transfected with pBR322 and Herpes simplex virus thymidine kinase (HSV tk) gene DNA.

40) [A26374] M.musculus HSV thymidine kinase 5′ non coding region.

14 PCR Protocols in Molecular Toxicology

Several very similar entries have been removed for brevity of text, however it should be apparent that the vast majority of these entries are not what is desired. In fact, the output could have been somewhat more abbreviated if the search had been:

"thymidine kinase" AND (mice OR mouse) NOT virus

Nonetheless, by perusing the list one can pick up [MUSTKM] as the most likely candidate for the wild-type genomic sequence. To retrieve this sequence, send the following message:

```
From: your.address@your.institution
Date: 2 Jan 1997 21:29:02-EDT
To: retrieve@ncbi.nlm.nih.gov
Subject: TK Sequence
DATALIB genbank
MAXDOCS 300
MAXLINES 2000
TITLES
BEGIN
MUSTKM [LOC]
```

The reply from GenBank then is:

```
Date: 24-Nov-96 20:30 EST
From: RETRIEVE E-Mail Server > your.address@your.institution
Subj: Results-RETRIEVE Server:tk

=================================================================
Database: GenBank Updates (89.0+, 07/05/95)
Query: mustkm [loc]
Parse status: OK: 0 documents retrieved.
Parse status: OK: 0 documents retrieved.
//
Database: GenBank (89.0, 6/9/95)
Query: mustkm [loc]
Parse status: OK: 1 document retrieved.
Documents selected: 1 (up to 2000 lines)
LOCUS   MUSTKM   2939 bp   DNA      ROD   24-SEP-1992
DEFINITION   Mouse thymidine kinase gene, complete cds.
ACCESSION   M68489
KEYWORDS   thymidine kinase.
SOURCE   Mouse (strain C57BL/10J) liver DNA, clone Mtk116.
  ORGANISM Mus musculus
     Eukaryota; Animalia; Chordata; Vertebrata; Mammalia; Theria;
     Eutheria; Rodentia; Myomorpha; Muridae; Murinae.
REFERENCE   1 (bases 1 to 2939)
AUTHORS Gudas,J.M., Fridovich-Keil,J.L., Datta,M.W., Bryan,J. and
     Pardee,A.B.
```

The Basics of the Polymerase Chain Reaction

```
TITLE   Characterization of the murine thymidine kinase-encoding gene and
   analysis of transcription start point heterogeneity
JOURNAL   Gene 118, 205-216 (1992)
MEDLINE   92380505
COMMENT
   NCBI gi: 202078
FEATURES        Location/Qualifiers
   source      1..2939
        /organism="Mus musculus"
        /strain="C57BL/10J"
        /sequenced_mol="DNA"
        /tissue_type="liver"
   mRNA      join(1..238,320..351,844..954,1180..1273,1496..1585,
        1737..1856,2162..2775)
        /gene="thymidine kinase"
        /product="thymidine kinase"
   exon      1..238
        /gene="thymidine kinase"
        /number=1
   protein_bind 77..85
        /bound_moiety="Sp1"
   CDS      join(173..238,320..351,844..954,1180..1273,1496..1585,
        1737..1856,2162..2350)
        /gene="thymidine kinase"
        /note="NCBI gi: 202079"
        /codon_start=1
        /product="thymidine kinase"
        /translation="MSYINLPTVLPSSPSKTRGQIQVILGPMFSGKSTELMRRVRRFQ
        IAQYKCLVIKYAKDTRYSNSFSTHDRNTMDALPACMLRDVTQEALGVAVIGI
        DEGQFF PDIVDFCEMMANEGKTVIVAALDGTFQRKAFGSILNLVPLAESV
        VKLTAVCMECFREA AYTKRLGLEKEVEVIGGADKYHSVCRLC
        YFKKSSAQTAGSDNKNCLVLGQPGEALVVR KLFASQQVLQYNSAN"
   intron      239..319
        /gene="thymidine kinase"
        /number=1
   exon 2162..2775
        /gene="thymidine kinase"
        /number=7
   polyA_signal 2755..2760
        /gene="thymidine kinase"
BASE COUNT 641 a 883 c 742 g 673 t
ORIGIN
   1 ccatggcaga tccggaggga tggtcgagct ccaggctttt cacgtagctg agaggtggga
  61 cgagtcttgt cttcgtcccg cccccttttg agttcgcggg caaatgcgag cagtaagtcg
 121 aaattttccc acccacggac tctcggtgct aactaaggtt tgcacagcag ccatgagcta
. . . . .
2761 gtttactact aatgagaacg tgtttctcct tagcctgggt ttccctaact tgcaaccggc
2821 acccacatga cttggggggta gaaatgtgtt ttgtagtacc aatggtctca ccacagccca
2881 agaagaacag tcccccacat ttctatctgg ttggtttcgt gacaaaaaat ggcaaagaa
//
```

Again, this return message has been edited for brevity.

The message must next be saved to a text file. Instructions for this operation would be unique to the particular electronic mail program being used.

Finally, to be useful for many programs the "header" information must be edited out of this file. This is all the addressing and search information at the start of the file up to, but not including, the line that starts with "LOCUS MUSTKM 2939 bp . . .". This editing operation can be accomplished with either a text editor, such as Notepad (MS-Windows) or TeachText (Macintosh), or a standard word processing program such as WordPerfect or Word. In the latter case, however, the edited file must be saved in the "text only" format. Text format is also referred to as ASCII, for American Standard Code For Information Interchange, a computer standard for representing upper and lower case letters, as well as numbers on a standard keyboard. Most word processors, however, store their files by default as binary files, which consist of eight-bit strings of data (versus seven-bit strings for ASCII). One must intentionally choose to save the file in text format, otherwise other programs for subsequently analyzing the GenBank sequence will not be able to use the file.

B.   Access to GenBank through the World Wide Web

Access to GenBank through the World Wide Web (WWW) offers some distinct advantages over access through Email. The WWW access offers three different interfaces, and setting up the search logic can be simpler. Furthermore, the results of a search can be almost immediate, allowing one to quickly modify the search if the desired result has not yet been obtained. On the other hand, the WWW can be notoriously slow (the fastest times are generally 6 to 9 a.m. EST on the weekends). Thus for relatively simple searches, or to retrieve a sequence for which one knows the locus name or accession number, retrieval through Email may be less frustrating.

Sites on the World Wide Web are accessed through browser software, the most popular being Netscape, Mosaic, and Microsoft Internet Explorer. For all browsers the general principles are the same: sites on the WWW are accessed by going to or opening a location or address called a URL (Uniform Resource Locator). A page is displayed and choices are selected by clicking with the mouse pointer on highlighted text.

To start the search for the mouse thymidine kinase gene sequence, we need to visit the Web site for NCBI. In Netscape click on the OPEN Icon; in Microsoft Internet Explorer click on the Open icon or the menu item File, Open and enter the address http://www.ncbi.nlm.nih.gov/. After clicking on OK or pressing Enter (and if the Internet connection is good) the screen shown in Figure 1.5 will appear.

As might be apparent from this home page, several approaches may be used to search GenBank. The approach described here makes use of the Entrez interface, which can retrieve a variety of information. To access, click on the *Entrez* button at the top of Web page. The page will look similar to Figure 1.6.

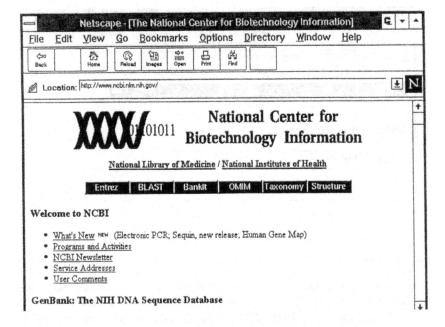

Figure 1.5
Netscape screen.

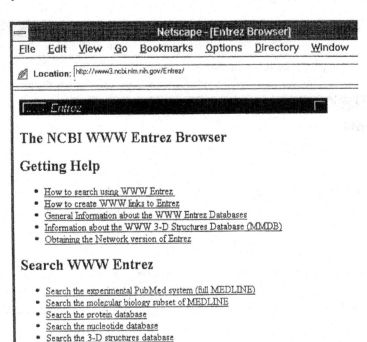

Figure 1.6
First Entrez screen.

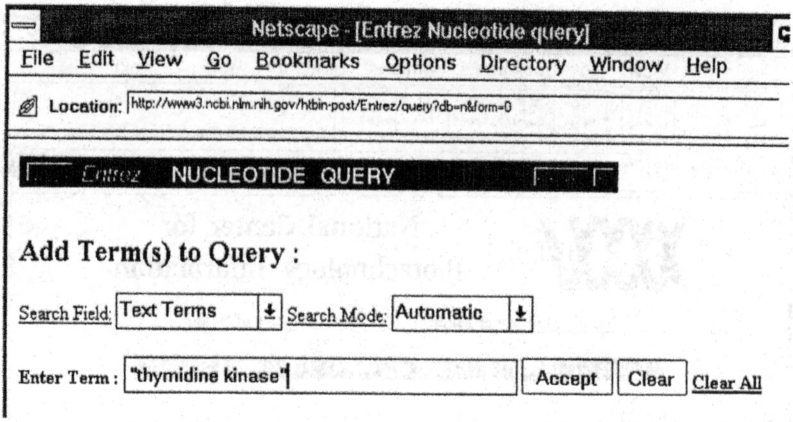

18   PCR Protocols in Molecular Toxicology

Figure 1.7
Entrez Nucleotide search screen.

Under *Search WWW Entrez*, click with the mouse on "Search the nucleotide database." The page that will be presented is seen in Figure 1.7.

Position the cursor in the *Enter Term* box and type the first term (or in this case, phrase, enclosed in quotes) in the appropriate box. Click *Accept* and the results seen in Figure 1.8 are presented.

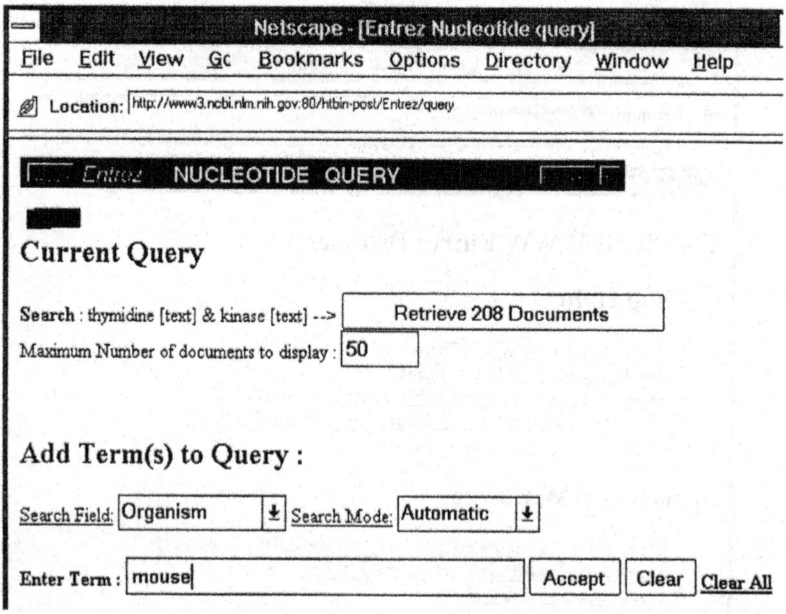

Figure 1.8
Entrez results 1.

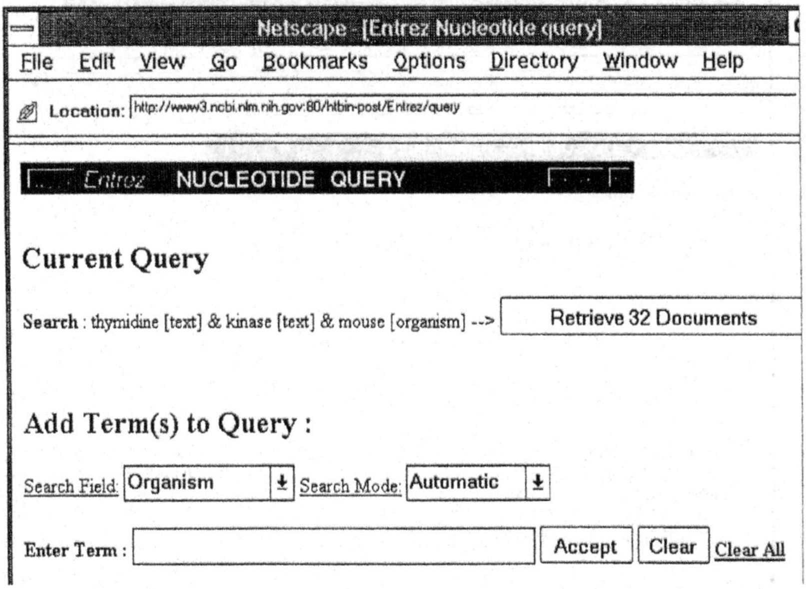

The Basics of the Polymerase Chain Reaction

19

```
┌────────────────────────────────────────────────────────────────────┐
│ ─         Netscape - [Entrez Nucleotide query]                     ( │
│ File   Edit   View   Go   Bookmarks   Options   Directory   Window   Help │
│ ──────────────────────────────────────────────────────────────────── │
│  🖉  Location: http://www3.ncbi.nlm.nih.gov:80/htbin-post/Entrez/query │
│ ──────────────────────────────────────────────────────────────────── │
│                                                                      │
│   ┌──  Entrez  NUCLEOTIDE QUERY              ┌─ ─ ┌                  │
│                                                                      │
│   Current Query                                                      │
│                                                                      │
│   Search : thymidine [text] & kinase [text] & mouse [organism] -->  ┌──────────────────────┐ │
│                                                                     │  Retrieve 32 Documents │ │
│                                                                     └──────────────────────┘ │
│                                                                      │
│   Add Term(s) to Query :                                            │
│                                                                      │
│   Search Field: │Organism        │ ⬍│ Search Mode: │Automatic   │ ⬍│ │
│                                                                      │
│   Enter Term : │                                    │ │ Accept │ │ Clear │ Clear All │
└────────────────────────────────────────────────────────────────────┘
```

Figure 1.9
Entrez results 2.

This Web page indicates that the search has identified 208 entries, far too many to visually scan for the proper one. To narrow the search (i.e., "Add Term(s) to Query:") click on the down arrow next to the *Search Field* box and highlight the field *Organism*. Then click in the box for "Enter Term:" and type mouse. Finally click on the box *Accept* to start the modified search.

The screen shown in Figure 1.9 will be displayed. The box "Retrieve 32 Documents" indicates that a manageable number of entries were found. Click on this box and the list of entries is displayed (Figure 1.10). Obviously this is just the top of the list and if one scrolls through it, one can find the entry MUSTKM (M68489). The short definition of this entry indicates that it is the complete coding sequence (cds) for the gene (i.e., genomic sequence). Complementary DNA (cDNA) sequences are indicated as such or as mRNA.

Following the entry is the line (View GenBank format, Report format, FASTA format, ASN.1 format, Graphical view, or Save As...). Clicking on *GenBank format* retrieves the screen shown in Figure 1.11. Examining the text here confirms that this is the desired entry. It clearly contains the sequence and information for the entire gene, although one must scroll through this entry to view all the information.

To save this data as a file on one's own computer for subsequent analysis, click on the box *Save As* ... which is at the top of the Web page. The "Saving Reports" Web page is presented. Click on the *Save as* button at the top and a window will appear similar to the one seen in Figure 1.12. This window will be specific for different browser programs, but the important features will be

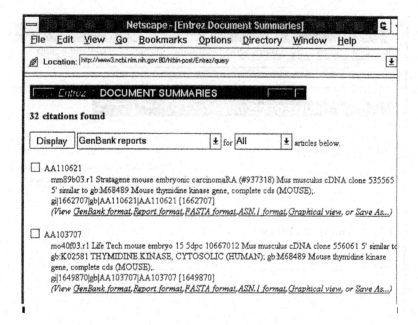

Figure 1.10
Entrez results list.

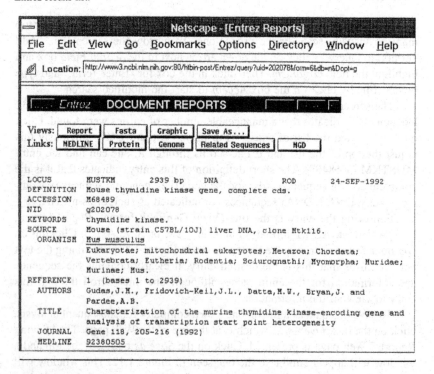

Figure 1.11
GenBank format in Entrez.

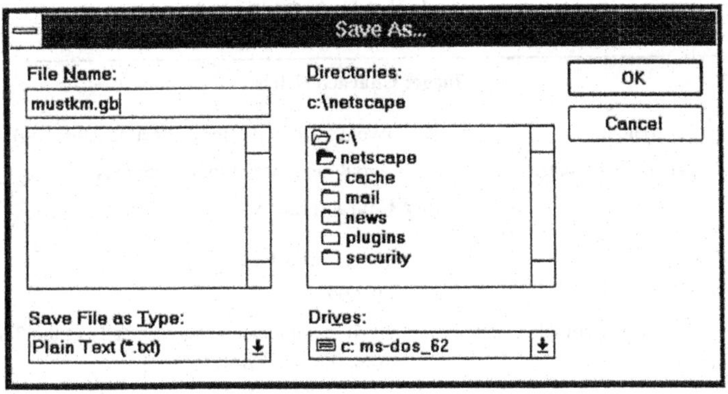

The Basics of the Polymerase Chain Reaction   **21**

Figure 1.12
Saving GenBank file.

similar. Make a note of the directory or folder where the file is being saved and the name given, and most important, **save the file as Plain Text**. When the *OK* button is clicked, the file will be transferred from GenBank to your computer. Our tour of the Web is done.

IV.   Primer Design

A.   Primer Characteristics

In the experience of this and many other laboratories, the single most important component of a successful PCR project is a set of carefully designed oligonucleotide primers. No other factor, save for contamination, has such an impact. And while several primer sets can empirically be compared, it is probably more cost-effective to carefully select the oligonucleotide primers based on their thermodynamic characteristics. The critical characteristics of successful PCR primers are listed in Table 1.2.

Several perspectives guide the design of primers, the first of which is the target to be amplified. The target region should be checked for its intra-strand complementarity, i.e., its ability to form stable hairpin structures that would interfere with the progress of DNA polymerase. In addition, the GC content of the target (and the PCR product) should be examined, as well as its predicted Tm. Targets with high GC contents (>70%) may require denaturation times greater than 1 min at 95°, and if such conditions are considered, so should DNA polymerases even more thermostable than *Taq* (e.g., *Pfu*, Vent, Deep Vent, etc.).

Primers themselves should have average GC content (40 to 60% G+C), but far more critical are the characteristics controlled by their DNA sequence. If primers have sequences that can form duplexes either within the same molecule or with the other primer, and these duplexes are greater than 3 or

TABLE 1.2
Characteristics of Successful PCR Primers

Target Characteristics	
Target GC content	Avoid >70% GC (may affect denaturation)
Target secondary structure	Avoid intra-strand loops, hairpins

Primer Characteristics	
Primer length	15–30 bases long
G+C content	40–60%
Inter-, intra-primer complementary	Avoid complementarity, especially at the 3' ends (i.e., Primer Dimer!!)
Internal secondary structure (hairpins)	Avoid stable hairpins
Homopolymer sequences (runs)	Avoid long stretches of any one base
Tm range	55 to 80°C
Specificity at 3' end	Terminal 7 bases must be specific
Internal vs. 3' terminal stability	3' ends should be least stable portion of primer

4 bases, than the primers themselves (which are at high concentration) will compete with the template for hybridization sites. If these complementary regions are at the 3' ends of the primers, DNA polymerase will catalyze the formation of what is called "primer dimer," and all primers will be tied up in such products in just a few cycles. This ability of DNA polymerase to make use of just the 3' end of the primer also requires that the bases at the 3' end be very specific, certainly within the DNA target being amplified. Thus, it is a good practice to check the terminal 7 bases at the 3' end for other sites of homology on the target. If there are such sites, choose a different sequence for a primer. Likewise, to drive the overall specificity of the primer, its 3' end should be the least stable portion of the oligonucleotide. The net effect of this design is that at stringent annealing temperatures the internal portion will form a duplex first, with the 3' terminus forming a duplex (and hence priming) only on the specific sequence.

Obviously, the process of examining short segments of DNA sequence for potential primers with the desired characteristics is precisely the sort of task suited to computer software. There are more than a dozen software packages, most commercially available, that allow automatic design of PCR primers, and for the purposes of this chapter the use of two will be described. The first, OLIGO®, developed by Wojciech Rychlik,[12] is one of the most expensive programs, yet it considers a large number of factors in primer design. The second program, PRIMER, by S.E. Lincoln, M.J. Daly, and E.S. Lander of the Whitehead Institute, is available for no charge over the Internet from its authors. Both programs are extensively documented, so the exercises given here will only serve as general examples. In this discussion the terms 5' primer, upper primer, or forward primer will be used interchangeably, as will 3' primer, lower primer, or reverse primer.

The Basics of the Polymerase Chain Reaction **23**

B.　Primer Design Using OLIGO® Software

The OLIGO program is available from National Biosciences, Inc., for Macintosh as well as MS-Windows packages, so its interface follows reasonably common conventions. GenBank files are directly read by the OLIGO program, so by using the File, Open command, the downloaded file (MUSTKM.gb in our example) can be accessed. The sequence is displayed, as well as a graph of melting temperature (Tm) values for oligonucleotide segments. Primer pairs may be automatically designed using the *Search, For Primers,* and *Probes* command.

The *Primers* and *Probes* search allows settings of several critical parameters (see Figure 1.13), but for a simple search the default parameters can be used, and one only need set the *Search Ranges.* For this example, the target region chosen will be exons 3 through 5 of the mouse *tk* gene, bases 844 to 1585. The *Search Ranges* will be set to 800 to 1200 for the *Positive Strand Primer* search and 1200 to 1600 for the *Negative Strand Primer* search. Setting the PCR product length to 400 to 800 completes the settings. Clicking on OK in the *Search for Primers* window starts the routines, which on a fast computer may take a minute or two.

The results window indicates that 253 pairs were accepted. To display this list, click on *Primer pairs.* The list also indicates for each pair the length, predicted "optimal" annealing temperature (Ta), and %GC of the PCR product (see Table 1.3). Obviously the position of the primer pairs can be used as a

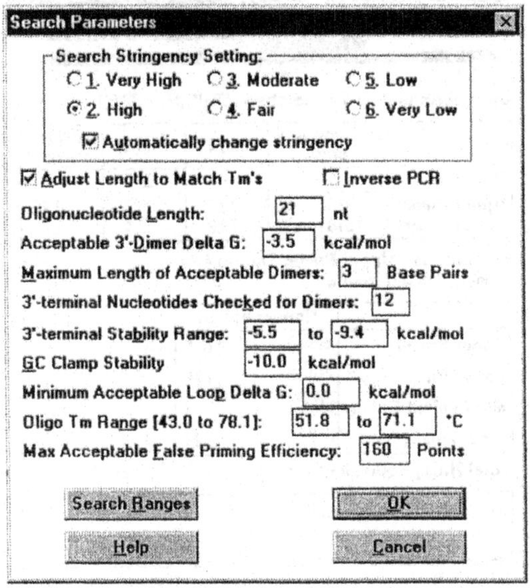

Figure 1.13
OLIGO input — PCR primer search parameters.

TABLE 1.3
OLIGO Output — Partial List of Acceptable PCR Primers

#	Positions of Primers	Prod.	Len	Opt. Ta	%GC
1	181	1303	513	60.4	54.2
2	812	1302	511	59.8	54.2
3	812	1303	512	60.3	54.3
4	813	1302	509	58.8	54.0
5	813	1303	509	58.6	54.0
6	813	1518	726	59.0	53.6
7	815	1539	745	56.7	53.3
8	898	1217	336	56.0	52.7

criterion for selection, but a high optimal annealing temperature can be an indication that the primer set could work under stringent conditions and be suited for high specificity. When a given primer pair is highlighted with the mouse, more calculated values for the PCR are displayed, as shown in Figure 1.14. More specifics on the primers themselves, including their sequence, are given in the *Window, Selected Primers* command.

One calculation carried out by OLIGO that is of particular interest is the *False Priming Sites* command, under the *Analyze* menu (see also reference 13). This procedure calculates a "priming efficiency" for a given primer at

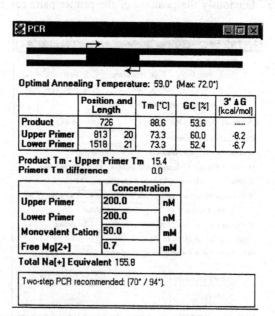

Figure 1.14
OLIGO output — PCR parameters.

The Basics of the Polymerase Chain Reaction

```
MUSTKM.GBX        Length:2939
Upper Primer False Priming Sites

UPPER PRIMER -- positive strand.
Priming efficiency of the perfect match is 463 (above the threshold).
Priming efficiency: 120.
5'(813)       GGGCCTCATGTGCTCT-GGTT (832)3'
              |||||| || || ||| ||||
3'(2365)   tccggagtccaggggagtcaa (2345)5'
Priming efficiency: 69.
5'(813)       GGGCCTCATGTGCTCTGGTT (832)3'
              | ||||| || |||| |
3'(2569)   acaggagtg---gaaaccga (2553)5'
Priming efficiency: 45.
5'(813)       GGGCCTCATGTGCTCTGGTT (832)3'
                |||||||| || ||
3'(596)      atgggggtacaccaggcgga (577)5'
Priming efficiency: 37.
5'(813)       GGGCCTCATGTGCTCTGGTT (832)3'
                || ||| || ||| |||||
3'(2840)   atgggggttcagtacaccca (2821)5'
---------------------------------------------------------------
UPPER PRIMER -- negative strand.
Priming efficiency of the perfect match is 463 (above the threshold).
Priming efficiency: 463 (above the threshold).
5'(813)       GGGCCTCATGTGCTCTGGTT (832)3'
              ||||||||||||||||||||
3'(813)    cccggagtacacgagaccaa (832)5'
Priming efficiency: 158.
5'(813)       GGGCCTCATGTGC-TCTGGTT (832)3'
                ||| |||| ||||||||
3'(2892)   gggggtgtaaagatagaccaa (2912)5'
Priming efficiency: 96.
5'(813)       GGGCCTCATGTGCTCTGGTT (832)3'
                || ||| || |||||||
3'(1979)   acccgaat-c-cgagaccga (1996)5'
Priming efficiency: 64.
5'(813)       GGGCCTCATGTGCTCTGGTT (832)3'
                |          ||||||||
3'(1587)   attctacagactgagaccga (1606)5'
```

Figure 1.15
OLIGO output — false priming sites.

possible false priming sites on both strands and is a test for specificity at the 3' terminus of the primer (see Figure 1.15). This calculation is critical if one is checking existing primers for potential problems, or choosing a primer outside the program's automatic search function.

Related to false priming is the issue of internal versus 3' terminal stability for a primer. OLIGO displays a plot of internal stability defined as the delta G values for 5-base oligonucleotide segments within a larger oligonucleotide primer. If the 3' terminus of a primer is the most stable part of the molecule, then the entire oligonucleotide need not completely anneal to prime synthesis, i.e., it causes polymerization at sites other than the target. The internal stability of forward and reverse primers can be checked with the *Analyze, Internal Stability* command.

As noted above, the target sequence itself, i.e., the PCR product, should be checked for extremely stable hairpin loops, but this operation is not directly offered by OLIGO. Rather the approach is to set the position of the *Current Oligo* to the start of the PCR product, then change the oligo length to that of the PCR product. In our example, that would entail changing the start position to 813 and the oligo length to 726 base pairs. Using *Analyze, Hairpin Formation, Current Oligo*, the PCR product may be scanned for hairpins. Loops with a ΔG stability of <-11 kcal/mol are probably a sign that the template has

26 PCR Protocols in Molecular Toxicology

some GC-rich regions and may require more aggressive denaturation conditions and/or an additive such as DMSO or formamide.

C.   Primer Design Using PRIMER

PRIMER (version 0.5) can be obtained at one of the Whitehead Institute's World Wide Web sites: http://www.genome.wi.mit.edu/ftp/distribution/software/primer.0.5/. Not only are the program files for Macintosh and MS-DOS present, but also the documentation files and source code so that the program could be compiled to run on any computer; the authors request that all files be downloaded. A more advanced version (3.0) of the program is available for SPARC stations.

PRIMER requires a particular sequence file format as outlined in its documentation. The GenBank file should be edited to replace all text preceding the sequence with the line:

*sequence: Mustkm

which indicates that a new sequence is following. For this exercise, a second line is inserted preceding the sequence, reading:

*subsequence: 801-1600

indicating to PRIMER that only this region will be examined. Other commands are possible and are noted in the documentation for the program.

The program runs at the MS-DOS command line, or in a Macintosh command window, and once started, prompts the user for information, such as the sequence file, the output file, and the file for any previously stored search criteria. Note that the region to be examined may be indicated as a "subsequence" or as a "target," with somewhat different results, but that this information is not prompted for, and must be inserted in the sequence file. The program gives the choice of automatic primer searches or manual testing of primers. With the automatic primer search the program prompts for the parameters indicated in Figure 1.16, offering default values in lieu of input.

The results of the search are stored in a file, in this case named MUSTKM.PCR (Figure 1.17). In fact, during the search the program indicated that the region examined, and hence the number of forward and reverse primers, was too large, so in fact the search was limited at 500 forward and 500 reverse primers. Only one primer pair is given for each product size range, and it should be noted that the numbering of the primer sequences is relative to the region examined, not to the original sequence (i.e., forward primer 14→33 corresponds to bases 814 to 833 in MUSTKM). PRIMER does not carry out a calculation for "optimal annealing temperature," but reports the Tm's for

The Basics of the Polymerase Chain Reaction

```
File containing PRIMER criteria
[hit RETURN to enter new criteria now]:

OPTIMAL primer length [20]:
MINIMUM primer length [18]:
MAXIMUM primer length [22]: 24
OPTIMAL primer melting temperature [60.0]: 62
MINIMUM acceptable primer melting temperature [57.0]:
MAXIMUM acceptable primer melting temperature [63.0]: 68
MINIMUM acceptable primer GC% [20]:
MAXIMUM acceptable primer GC% [80]:
Salt concentration (mM) [50.0]:
DNA concentration (nM) [50.0]:
MAXIMUM number of unknown bases (Ns) allowed in a primer [0]:
MAXIMUM acceptable primer self-complementarity (number of bases) [12]:
MAXIMUM acceptable 3' end primer self-complementarity (number of bases) [8]: 7
GC clamp how many 3' bases [0]:
Restriction sites which flank region of interest [ <none> ]:
Product length ranges [ 100-150 150-250 250-400 ]: 400-500 501-600 601-700 701-800
```

Figure 1.16
PRIMER input — PCR primer search parameters.

both primers. If an alternative primer set is desired, such a pair can be selected from the files of forward and reverse primers generated by the program; this pair can be checked with the program for acceptability.

```
*****************************************************************
* Output from:                                                  *
*                                                               *
*                          PRIMER                               *
*                       (Version 0.5)                           *
*                                                               *
*      Copyright 1991, Whitehead Institute for Biomedical Research  *
*****************************************************************


Analyzing sequence 1 (MUSTKM)

Acceptable regions for a primer:
base 1 to 800

Examining 781 forward primers...500 forward primers accepted.
Examining 781 reverse primers...500 reverse primers accepted.
Testing pairs...

Product size range 400-500...
forward primer   153->172 : CGGTCAGTCCTACCCCTGAG        Tm = 62.0
reverse primer   589->570 : TATAGGGCGAATTGGATCCG        Tm = 62.0
PCR product length:  437, GC = 54%

Product size range 501-600...
forward primer    78->97  : ATCGCCCAGTACAAGTGCCT        Tm = 62.0
reverse primer   589->570 : TATAGGGCGAATTGGATCCG        Tm = 62.0
PCR product length:  512, GC = 53%

Product size range 601-700...
forward primer    14->33  : GGCCTCATGTGCTCTGGTTA        Tm = 61.2
reverse primer   620->601 : CAAACGACGCCAGTGATTGT        Tm = 62.1
PCR product length:  607, GC = 53%

Product size range 701-800...
No acceptable pairs found!
```

Figure 1.17
PRIMER output — PCR primer search file.

D. Primer Design Using PRIMER 3.0, World Wide Web Version

As a final note, PRIMER version 3.0 is available for use over the World Wide Web, i.e., all that is needed here is an Internet connection! The parameters available exceed those in PRIMER version 0.5, and are entered or changed with the usual graphic World Wide Web form-based interface. Documentation is available online. The DNA sequence must be only sequence data, i.e., numbers will interfere with the analysis. Thus in the example of the MUSTKM file, not only must all header information be removed, but the sequence numbering must be eliminated as well. However, once that is done, the sequence is simply highlighted, copied to the Windows or Macintosh clipboard, and after switching to the Web browser at the PRIMER 3 site, pasted into the Source Sequence input box. The site for PRIMER 3 is:

http://www-genome.wi.mit.edu/cgi-bin/primer/primer3.cgi

As in the above example using PRIMER version 0.5, the *Included Region* was chosen as 801 to 1600, (designated as 801, 800 in the input form), with a *Product Size Range* of 200 to 800. The *Pick Primers* button is clicked, and the program returns the results shown in Figure 1.18.

E. Primer Synthesis

While some laboratories have access to a central oligonucleotide synthesis facility, most will rely on the vast number of companies that specialize in oligonucleotide synthesis. Prices are generally less than $1 per base, making two 20-base primers very affordable. Most companies deliver custom synthesized primers in a matter of days, with orders made by Fax or electronic mail to minimize errors of sequence transcription. Generally, deprotected and desalted quality oligonucleotides are quite suitable for PCR as is. Simply dissolve the oligonucleotide in sterile water to a concentration of 100 μM, aliquot, then dilute one of the aliquots to 20 μM for use in PCR. Store all aliquots at $-20°C$.

V. PCR Procedure and Optimization

A. Basic Considerations

Once primers have been obtained, optimal PCR conditions need to be determined, that is, the *yield* (the amount of desired PCR product), *specificity* (the

The Basics of the Polymerase Chain Reaction

```
Primer3 Output

Using 1-based sequence positions
OLIGO           start  len      tm    gc%    any    3' seq
LEFT PRIMER      943   20    59.96  55.00  6.00  3.00 cacacatgatcggtcagtcc
RIGHT PRIMER    1494   20    60.04  50.00  3.00  0.00 tgggaaaagtccagaggatg
SEQUENCE SIZE: 2939
INCLUDED REGION SIZE: 800

PRODUCT SIZE: 552, PAIR ANY COMPL: 3.00, PAIR 3' COMPL: 3.00

ADDITIONAL OLIGOS
                 start  len      tm    gc%    any    3' seq

1 LEFT PRIMER      943   20    59.96  55.00  6.00  3.00 cacacatgatcggtcagtcc
  RIGHT PRIMER    1161   20    59.96  55.00  2.00  1.00 gaatgagcaagggcagagac
  PRODUCT SIZE: 219, PAIR ANY COMPL: 4.00, PAIR 3' COMPL: 2.00

2 LEFT PRIMER      943   20    59.96  55.00  6.00  3.00 cacacatgatcggtcagtcc
  RIGHT PRIMER    1170   20    59.96  50.00  4.00  0.00 gaaggccaagaatgagcaag
  PRODUCT SIZE: 228, PAIR ANY COMPL: 4.00, PAIR 3' COMPL: 2.00

3 LEFT PRIMER      943   20    59.96  55.00  6.00  3.00 cacacatgatcggtcagtcc
  RIGHT PRIMER    1171   20    59.96  45.00  4.00  0.00 agaaggccaagaatgagcaa
  PRODUCT SIZE: 229, PAIR ANY COMPL: 4.00, PAIR 3' COMPL: 3.00

4 LEFT PRIMER     1142   20    59.96  55.00  2.00  0.00 gtctctgcccttgctcattc
  RIGHT PRIMER    1494   20    60.04  50.00  3.00  0.00 tgggaaaagtccagaggatg
  PRODUCT SIZE: 353, PAIR ANY COMPL: 6.00, PAIR 3' COMPL: 3.00

Statistics
          con   too    in    in            no    tm    tm   high  high
          sid  many   tar  excl   bad     GC   too   too    any    3'   poly
         ered    Ns   get   reg   GC% clamp   low  high compl compl     X     ok
Left     5941     0     0     0     0     0  1017  2089    15   955     0   1865
Right    5864     0     0     0     0     0  1033  2181    23   867     0   1760
Pair Stats:
considered 20, unacceptable product size 8, high end compl 3, ok 9
primer3 release 0.3
```

Figure 1.18
PRIMER 3.0 output — PCR primer search file.

ratio of desired product to that of nontarget products), and *fidelity* (the sequence accuracy of desired PCR product). Yield is essentially the efficiency of the PCR, but often the conditions favoring greatest specificity result in a reduced yield, so it is a balance between these goals that must be achieved. How the various parameters in a PCR affect these goals is summarized in Table 1.4. First and foremost is primer design, which has been discussed. Aggressive denaturation conditions, long extension times, and the use of a very thermostable DNA polymerase (e.g., Vent, *Pfu*) can be anticipated by the GC content, hairpin structure, and Tm of the template or target sequence.[14,15] Likewise, the use of a DNA polymerase with fidelity greater than that of *Taq* polymerase (e.g., Vent, *Pfu*) is dictated by the demands of the experiment: will the PCR product be cloned and, if so, what tolerance for error is allowed? Other parameters must be determined empirically, and this process should be done in a focused, methodical fashion because some parameters interact with others (e.g., free Mg^{2+} concentration is dependent upon deoxyribonucleotide (dNTP) concentration).

30 PCR Protocols in Molecular Toxicology

TABLE 1.4
Parameters Affecting Basic Goals of PCR

Parameter	Yield	Specificity	Fidelity
Primer Design	X	X	
Denaturation	X		X
Annealing	X	X	
Extension	X		
DNA Polymerase	X	X	X
[Mg^{++}]	X	X	X
[dNTP]	X		X
[primer]	X	X	
[target]	X	X	
Additives	X	X	

B. Basic Protocol for Oil-Overlay Thermocyclers

Note: *The protocol for oil-overlay thermocyclers is slightly different than for heated-lid models, the main difference being the inclusion of a drop of mineral oil per tube in the former case. The oil overlay will prevent evaporation of sample during the PCR as will the heated lid (100°C) in the newer models. The only other parameter that is different between the two types of thermocyclers is the times per cycle. Generally, the time required at each step (denaturing, annealing, and elongation) are twice as long in the oil-overlay models. The optimization steps discussed below may be performed with these caveats in mind.*

Essentially a master mix is prepared, then aliquoted to individual reaction tubes.

Number of reactions →	6	Multiplication factor →	6.5
Total Rx Volume	50 µl	Sample Size	10

- Prepare in order

			Concentrations		
Totals	Component		Initial	Final	Per rx
1. 187.53 µl	Sterile DI water				28.9 µl
2. 32.50 µl	10X Rx buffer	Lot-_____	10	1 X	5.0 µl
3. 19.50 µl	MgCl	Lot-_____	25	1.5 mM	3.0 µl

The Basics of the Polymerase Chain Reaction

•	Vortex					
4. 2.60 µl	dNTPs (Mixed)	Lot-_____	25	0.2 mM	0.4 µl
5. 8.13 µl	Upstream Primer	Lot-_____	20	0.5 µM	1.25 µl
6. 8.13 µl	Downstream Primer	Lot-_____	20	0.5 µM	1.25 µl
7. 1.63 µl	*Taq* polymerase	Lot-_____	500	2.5u/100µl	0.3 µl

- Triturate to mix
- Aliquot 40 µl of the master mix into individual reaction tubes
- Add 10 µl of DNA sample to each tube. (See below for optimization of DNA concentration.)
- Include at least one negative control tube (i.e., no DNA) with either 10 µl buffer or sterile water
- Overlay each reaction mixture with a drop of mineral oil (e.g., Sigma Cat # M-5904).
- After thermocycling, transfer 10 µl of each PCR mix to a tube containing 2.5 µl 5X gel loading buffer and carry out electrophoresis as described in Chapter 6.

C.   DNA Sample for Optimization

The sample used for the optimization experiments should be a high-quality DNA preparation known to contain the target sequence. For initial optimization start with adding 10^5 copies to each reaction (see Table 1.5).

D.   Optimization Experiment 1 — Cycle Number

As noted above (see also Figure 1.3), if the PCR is carried out to the point of plateau, differences between samples in terms of starting number of copies, or efficiency of amplification, will be masked. Thus, the first experiment in optimization is to get a crude estimate of the number of amplification cycles that yield enough product to be visualized with ethidium bromide staining.

TABLE 1.5
Sizes of Various Genomes and Copies per Microgram

	bp	Daltons	Copies/µg	µg/10^5	µg/10^6
Plasmid	5.00E+03	3.25E+06	1.86E+11	5.39E–07	5.39E–06
E. coli	4.70E+06	3.05E+09	1.97E+08	5.07E–04	5.07E–03
Mouse	2.70E+09	1.75E+12	3.44E+05	0.29	2.91
Human	3.30E+09	2.14E+12	2.81E+05	0.36	3.56

32 PCR Protocols in Molecular Toxicology

One parameter, the annealing temperature, will have to be estimated. The optimal annealing temperature (Ta^{OPT}) calculated by the OLIGO program may be used; this is actually calculated according to the formula $Ta^{OPT} = 0.3 \times$ Tm(primer) + 0.7 × Tm(product) −14.9.[12] Alternatively one may use a formula determined by Wu et al., where Tm is calculated for each primer as 22 + 1.46 · {2 · (#G or C) + (#A or T)} and the lowest value is used for annealing.[16] The latter formula gives higher annealing temperatures than the former, but for the purposes of an initial experiment, either will do.

- Prepare five PCR mixtures with DNA sample
- Prepare one negative control (no DNA)
- Set thermocycler parameters to
  - One initial cycle at 95° for 4 min (to initially denature the sample)
  - 40 cycles:
    - 95° for 1 min
    - Calculated annealing temp (Ta^{CALC}) for 1 min
    - 72° for 1 min
- After 20 cycles (not counting the initial cycle) remove sample 1 and place on ice
- After 25 cycles remove sample 2, etc.
- Sample 5 and the negative control are given 40 cycles
- Electrophorese 5 μl of each PCR reaction on an agarose gel and stain with ethidium bromide as discussed in Chapter 6.

E. Optimization Experiment 2 — Annealing Temperature

An optimal annealing temperature is particularly important if PCR products are observed that are clearly not of the expected molecular weight. This experiment will be somewhat cumbersome, because it requires five separate thermocycler runs. (On the other hand, Stratagene produces a thermocycler that can accomplish this experiment with one run.)

- Prepare five PCR mixtures with sample
- Prepare one negative control (i.e., no DNA) — either buffer or sterile water
- Select the number of cycles X, based on which yielded a *reasonable* (but not maximal) amount of PCR products on a gel. (See above)
- For sample 1, the annealing temperature will be set to 8°C below the calculated annealing temperature used in experiment 1; thus the thermocycler parameters are:
  - One initial cycle at 95° for 4 min (to initially denature the sample)
  - X cycles at 95° for 1 min, (Ta^{CALC} − 8°C) for 1 min, 72° for 1 min

The Basics of the Polymerase Chain Reaction

- Other samples will be cycled with the same parameters except for the annealing temperature:
  - Sample 2 $Ta^{CALC} - 4°C$
  - Sample 3 and negative control Ta^{CALC}
  - Sample 4 $Ta^{CALC} + 4°C$
  - Sample 5 $Ta^{CALC} + 8°C$
- Store all samples on ice when not thermocycling
- Electrophorese 5 µl of each PCR reaction mix on an agarose gel and stain with ethidium bromide.

The desired annealing temperature is obviously the one that gives the greatest amount of desired product with the least amount of extraneous products. It is possible that a second round of annealing temperature optimization may be required, with either a narrower temperature range (e.g., 2°C increments) or a range farther away from the calculated annealing temperature. On the other hand, a "hot start" procedure should be tried first if extraneous products persist at all annealing temperatures in Optimization Experiment 2.

F.   Optimization Experiment 3 — Hot Start

As annealing temperature is reduced, duplexes between the primers and nontarget sequences become more stable. These duplexes are extended by *Taq* polymerase because this enzyme retains a fair amount of activity even at temperatures as low as 22°C,[17] and thus extraneous products almost certainly appear at these lower annealing temperatures. Yet such products have the opportunity to be formed even when the annealing temperature is quite high, since in the simplest PCR experiment the reaction mixture is heated from room temperature to the initial denaturation temperature, with a limited but finite time at temperatures in between. Several workers recognized that these initial opportunities for mispriming unbalanced the PCR from the start: the myriad of nontarget products generated from these events contain incorporated primer sequences, and hence could be replicated even under stringent conditions later in the PCR. These products not only show up as extraneous bands upon electrophoresis, but also reduce the yield of the target product through competition. The solution these workers proposed was to add a key reagent (e.g., *Taq* polymerase, or dNTPs) to the reaction mixture only after a temperature >70°C was reached[6,18] ("physical hot start"; for application of this type of hot start, see Chapter 2). This approach was later modified to separate a key component from the rest of the reaction by a wax barrier that melted only at high temperatures.[19] Perkin-Elmer markets AmpliWax® beads for such a wax-mediated HotStart™ technique. More recently, a monoclonal antibody has been developed (TaqStart™ from CLONTECH) that inactivates *Taq* polymerase at lower temperatures. At high temperatures it is itself inac-

34   PCR Protocols in Molecular Toxicology

tivated, and *Taq* polymerase begins DNA synthesis. For a vast number of PCR designs some sort of hot start improves specificity and yield, so it is worth examining its effect on a novel PCR. This example will describe the use of TaqStart, although a wax-mediated or physical hot start could be examined as an alternative.

Number of reactions →3 (for each mixture)   Multiplication factor →   3.5
Total Rx Volume   50 µl   Sample Size   10 µl

- Prepare "standard PCR," in order

Totals	Component		Initial	Final	Per rx
			Concentrations		
1. 100.98 µl	Sterile DI water				28.9 µl
2. 17.50 µl	10X Rx buffer	Lot-_____	10	1 X	5.0 µl
3. 10.50 µl	MgCl	Lot-_____	25	1.5 mM	3.0 µl
	• Vortex				
4. 1.40 µl	dNTPs (Mixed)	Lot-_____	25	0.2 mM	0.4 µl
5. 4.38 µl	Upstream Primer	Lot-_____	20	0.5 µM	1.25 µl
6. 4.38 µl	Downstream Primer	Lot-_____	20	0.5 µM	1.25 µl
7. 0.88 µl	*Taq* polymerase	Lot-_____	500	2.5u/100µl	0.3 µl

- Triturate to mix
- Aliquot 40 µl to reaction tubes 1 through 3
- Prepare "hot-start PCR," in order

Totals	Component		Initial	Final	Per rx
			Concentrations		
1. 3.50 µl	TaqStart Dil Buffer	Lot-_____			1.0 µl
2. 0.88 µl	TaqStart Antibody	Lot-_____	25	0.2	0.3 µl
	• Triturate to mix				
3. 0.88 µl	*Taq* polymerase	Lot-_____	500	2.5u/100 µl	0.3 µl
	• Triturate to mix				
	• Incubate >10 min at room temp				
4. 17.50 µl	10X Rx buffer	Lot-_____	10	1X	5.0 µl
5. 96.6 µl	Sterile DI water				27.6 µl
6. 10.50 µl	MgCl	Lot-_____	25	1.5 mM	3.0 µl
	• Vortex mix				

The Basics of the Polymerase Chain Reaction

7. 1.40 µl	dNTPs (Mixed)	Lot-_____	25	0.2 mM	0.4 µl
8. 4.38 µl	Upstream Primer	Lot-_____	20	0.5 µM	1.25 µl
9. 4.38 µl	Downstream Primer	Lot-_____	20	0.5 µM	1.25 µl

- Vortex to mix
- Aliquot 40 µl to reaction tubes 4 through 6
- Add 10 µl of DNA sample to tubes 1, 2, 4, and 5
- Add 10 µl of sterile water or buffer to tubes 3 and 6 (negative control)
- Overlay each reaction mixture with a drop of mineral oil (e.g., Sigma Cat # M-5904).
- Set thermocycler parameters to
  - One initial cycle at 95° for 4 min (to initially denature the sample)
  - X cycles (X is the number of cycles used in Experiment 2)
  - 95° for 1 min
  - Annealing temp determined in Experiment 2 for 1 min
  - 72° for 1 min
- After thermocycling, transfer 10 µl of each PCR mix to a tube containing 2.5 µl 5X gel loading buffer and carry out electrophoresis as described in Chapter 6.

G.   Optimization Experiment 4 — MgCl$_2$ Concentration

Optimizing the cycle number and annealing temperature, and determining the value of a hot-start procedure may be all that's necessary for a good PCR. On the other hand, many laboratories have found that small variations in the concentration of free Mg^{2+} ion in the reaction can have a profound effect on the quality and yield of a particular PCR. Free Mg^{2+} concentration is dependent upon not only added MgCl$_2$ but also the concentration of dNTPs. Furthermore, the optimal annealing temperature may be affected by the Mg^{2+} concentration. Thus a change in Mg^{2+} may necessitate a reoptimization of annealing conditions, and a change in dNTP concentration would warrant re-examining optimal Mg^{2+} concentration.

Number of reactions →6 (for each mixture)		Multiplication factor → 6.5		
Total Rx Volume 50 µl		Sample Size 10 µl		
• Prepare "hot-start PCR," in order				
			Concentrations	
Totals	Component	Initial	Final	Per rx
1. 6.50 µl	TaqStart Dil Buffer Lot-_____			1.0 µl

36 PCR Protocols in Molecular Toxicology

2. 1.63 µl	TaqStart Antibody	Lot-_____	25	0.2	0.3 µl
• Triturate to mix					
3. 1.63 µl	*Taq* polymerase	Lot-_____	500	2.5u/100µl	0.3 µl
• Triturate to mix					
• Incubate >10 min at room temp					
4. 32.50 µl	10X Rx buffer	Lot-_____	10	1X	5.0 µl
5. 146.90 µl	Sterile DI water				22.6 µl
6. 19.5 µl	MgCl	Lot-_____	25	1.5 mM	3.0 µl
• Vortex mix					
7. 2.60 µl	dNTPs (Mixed)	Lot-_____	25	0.2 mM	0.4 µl
8. 8.13 µl	Upstream Primer	Lot-_____	20	0.5 µM	1.25 µl
9. 8.13 µl	Downstream Primer	Lot-_____	20	0.5 µM	1.25 µl

- Vortex to mix
- Aliquot 35 µl to reaction tubes 1 through 6
- Add 10 µl of sample to tubes 1 through 5
- Add 10 µl of sterile water or buffer to tube 6
- Further additions:

  Tube 1   0 µl 25 mM MgCl$_2$ 5 µl sterile water   1.5 mM <u>total</u> Mg^{2+}

  Tube 2   1 µl 25 mM MgCl$_2$ 4 µl sterile water   2.0 mM

  Tube 3   2 µl 25 mM MgCl$_2$ 3 µl sterile water   2.5 mM

  Tube 4   3 µl 25 mM MgCl$_2$ 2 µl sterile water   3.0 mM

  Tube 5   4 µl 25 mM MgCl$_2$ 1 µl sterile water   3.5 mM

  Tube 6   0 µl 25 mM MgCl$_2$ 5 µl sterile water   1.5 mM

- Overlay each reaction mixture with a drop of mineral oil (e.g., Sigma Cat # M-5904).
- Set thermocycler parameters to
  - One initial cycle at 95° for 4 min (to initially denature the sample)
  - X cycles. (X is the number of cycles used in Experiment 2)
    - 95° for 1 min
    - Annealing temp determined in Experiment 2 – 1 min
    - 72° for 1 min
- After thermocycling, transfer 10 µl of each PCR mix to a tube containing 2.5 µl 5X gel loading buffer and carry out electrophoresis as described in Chapter 6.

The Basics of the Polymerase Chain Reaction

H. Additives and Other Optimization Approaches

Several laboratories have found that organic solvents can enhance the yield and specificity of PCR. Addition of 2 to 10% formamide has been shown to improve the yield and specificity of certain PCRs,[20-22] while 5% DMSO, 5 to 15% glycerol, and 5 to 15% PEG can also provide an enhancement.[23] Spermidine at 0.2 to 1 mM had an enhancing effect on PCR amplification of plant genomic sequences that was not seen with other additives.[24] Some commercially available additives (e.g., Perfect Match from Stratagene) may also provide a unique enhancement. Whether or not to use such additives is dictated by how poorly a given PCR is performing after optimizing parameters such as annealing temperature and Mg^{2+} concentration. In the case of GC-rich templates and/or those with secondary structure, such additions may provide an alternative to more aggressive denaturation conditions and a move to a thermostable DNA polymerase other than *Taq*.

Optimizing primer and dNTP concentrations also may be considered, but in the author's hands it is more critical with polymerases such as Vent or *Pfu* that have a 3′ to 5′ exonuclease function. As has been stated, varying the dNTP concentration has the effect of varying the free Mg^{2+} concentration, so both must be optimized in parallel.

Materials Needed

10X Rx Buffer

> 10X PCR Buffer II from Perkin Elmer (500 mM KCl; 100 mM Tris-HCl pH 8.3 at room temperature)

25 mM MgCl₂

25 mM mixed dNTPs

> Combine 100 μl each of 100 mM dATP, dCTP, dGTP, and dTTP (ultrapure solutions obtained from Pharmacia Biotech, # 27-2035-01)

PCR primers

> Custom synthesized, deprotected and desalted. Dissolve to 100 μM in sterile deionized water, and aliquot. Dilute one aliquot to a working solution of 20 μM.

Taq DNA polymerase

> Usually obtained at 5 units/μl

38   PCR Protocols in Molecular Toxicology

Light mineral oil
Molecular biology grade (e.g., Sigma Cat # M-5904)

TaqStart Antibody
From Clontech, #5400-1

References

1. **Mullis, K. B.,** The unusual origin of the polymerase chain reaction, *Sci. Am.*, 262, 56, 1990.
2. **Katz, E. D. and Haff, L. A.,** Effects of primer concentration and Taq DNA polymerase activity on yield of the PCR process, *Amplifications*, 3, 8, 1989.
3. **Sardelli, A. D.,** Plateau effect — understanding PCR limitations, *Amplifications*, 9, 1, 1993.
4. **Ferre, F.,** Quantitative or semi-quantitative PCR: reality vs. myth, *PCR Methods Applic.*, 2, 1, 1992.
5. **Murphy, L. D. et al.,** Use of the polymerase chain reaction in the quantitation of mdr-1 gene expression, *Biochemistry*, 29, 10351, 1990.
6. **Mullis, K. B.,** The polymerase chain reaction in an anemic mode: How to avoid cold oligodeoxyribonuclear fusion, *PCR Methods Applic.*, 1, 1, 1991.
7. **Dieffenbach, C. W. and Dveksler, G. S.,** Setting up a PCR laboratory, *PCR Methods Applic.*, 3, S2, 1993.
8. **Cone, R. W. and Fairfax, M. R.,** Protocol for ultraviolet irradiation of surfaces to reduce PCR contamination, *PCR Methods Applic.*, 3, S15, 1993.
9. **Hartley, J. L. and Rashtchian, A.,** Dealing with contamination: enzymatic control of carryover contamination in PCR, *PCR Methods Applic.*, 3, S10, 1993.
10. **Prince, A. M. and Andrus, L.,** PCR: how to kill unwanted DNA, *BioTechniques*, 12, 358, 1992.
11. **Bork, P. and Bairoch, A.,** Go hunting in sequence databases but watch out for the traps, *Trends Genet.*, 12, 425, 1996.
12. **Rychlik, W., Spencer, W. J., and Rhoads, R. E.,** Optimization of the annealing temperature for DNA amplification in vitro, *Nucleic Acids Res.*, 18, 6409, 1990.
13. **Rychlik, W.,** Priming efficiency in PCR, *BioTechniques*, 18, 84, 1995.
14. **Drummond, I. A. et al.,** Repression of the insulin-like growth factor II gene by the Wilms tumor suppressor WT1, *Science*, 257, 674, 1992.
15. **Dutton, C. M., Paynton, C., and Sommer, S. S.,** General method for amplifying regions of very high G+C content, *Nucleic Acids Res.*, 21, 2953, 1993.
16. **Wu, D. Y. et al.,** The effect of temperature and oligonucleotide primer length on the specificity and efficiency of amplification by the polymerase chain reaction, *DNA. Cell. Biol.*, 10, 233, 1991.
17. **Gelfand, D. H.,** in *PCR Technology* Erlich, H. A., Ed. Stockton Press, New York, 1989.
18. **D'Aquila, R. T. et al.,** Maximizing sensitivity and specificity of PCR by pre-amplification heating, *Nucleic Acids Res.*, 19, 3749, 1991.

19. **Chou, Q. et al.,** Prevention of pre-PCR mis-priming and primer dimerization improves low-copy-number amplifications, *Nucleic Acids Res.*, 20, 1717, 1992.
20. **Sarkar, G., Kapelner, S., and Sommer, S. S.,** Formamide can dramatically improve the specificity of PCR, *Nucleic Acids Res.*, 18, 7465, 1990.
21. **Comey, C. T., Jung, J. M., and Budowle, B.,** Use of formamide to improve amplification of HLA DQÂ sequences, *BioTechniques*, 10, 60, 1991.
22. **Schucard, M. et al.,** Two-step "hot" PCR amplification of GC-rich avian c-myc sequences, *BioTechniques*, 14, 390, 1993.
23. **Pomp, D. and Medrano, J. F.,** Organic solvents as facilitators of polymerase chain reaction, *BioTechniques*, 10, 58, 1991.
24. **Wan, C. Y. and Wilkins, T. A.,** Spermidine facilitates PCR amplification of target DNA, *PCR Methods Applic.*, 3, 208, 1993.

Chapter **2**

Analysis of Gene Expression

John P. Vanden Heuvel

Contents

I. General Strategies and Applications 42
II. Construction of Internal Standards 44
  A. Recombinant RNA Synthesis 45
    1. Basic Considerations 45
    2. Internal Standard Amplification 46
    3. *In Vitro* Transcription 47
  B. Low-Stringency Amplification 48
    1. Basic Considerations 48
    2. Internal Standard Amplification 49
  C. Amplification Across an Intron 50
    1. Basic Design 50
    2. Internal Standard Amplification 51
  D. Internal Standard with a Mutated Restriction
      Enzyme Site 52
    1. Basic Considerations 52
    2. Construction of PCR Cloning Vector 54
    3. Generation of Wild-Type Plasmid 55
    4. PCR Mutagenesis 57
  E. Testing Internal Standards 60
    1. Basic Considerations 60
    2. Amplification of a Dilution Series of rcRNA
        (Standard RT–PCR Procedures) 60

0-8493-3344-X/98/$0.00+$.50
© 1998 by CRC Press LLC

	3.	Amplification Efficiency of Internal Standard as Compared to the Target 63
III.	Competitive Quantitative RT–PCR.. 63	
	A.	General Competitive RT–PCR... 64
		1. Basic Considerations 64
		2. Constant Amount of RNA with Serial Dilutions of Internal Standard.. 65
		3. Quantitation 68
	B.	Quantitation Using a Standard Curve................................ 69
		1. Basic Considerations 69
		2. Competitive RT–PCR with Standard Curve 70
		3. Quantitation 73
IV.	Cycle-Based Quantitative RT–PCR.. 76	
	A.	Basic Considerations 76
	B.	Protocol... 77
		1. 5' Labeling of PCR Primer 77
		2. PCR Amplification 78
		3. Detection and Quantitation 81
V.	Semiquantitative RT–PCR 82	
	A.	Basic Considerations 82
	B.	Semiquantitative, External Standard RT–PCR 83
	C.	Quantitation 85
VI.	Reverse Transcription PCR In Situ Hybridization............................ 86	
	A.	Slide Preparation 86
	B.	cDNA Synthesis 86
	C.	PCR Amplification 87
	D.	Signal Detection 88
VII.	Analysis of Transcription Rate 89	
	A.	General Considerations 89
	B.	Protocol... 89
VIII.	Reporter Gene Analysis 91	
	A.	General Considerations 91
	B.	Protocol 1 91
	C.	Protocol 2 93
Reagents Needed.. 94		
References 96		

I. General Strategies and Applications

The examination of a particular treatment on gene expression is of fundamental interest to the molecular toxicologist.[1,2] Being able to explain not only which genes are affected but also attributing a particular mechanism (i.e., transcription versus mRNA stabilization) allows for a much broader understanding of the biological or toxicologic response. In this chapter we will detail how to

Analysis of Gene Expression

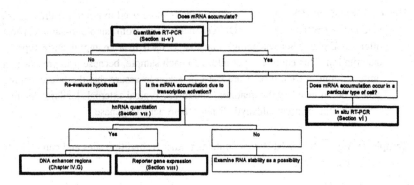

Figure 2.1
General strategies for analysis of gene expression utilizing polymerase chain reaction. The procedures that will be discussed in this chapter are highlighted.

utilize PCR to go from answering the fundamental question, "Does a particular treatment affect the expression of a gene of interest," to the examination of transcriptional activation, tissue distribution, and reporter gene analysis (see Figure 2.1).

Of course, the examination of mRNA accumulation can be determined in many cases by hybridization procedures such as Northern blots, dot- or slot-blots, and RNase protection assays. Each of these methods has distinct advantages and limitations when compared to its counterpart, PCR-based assays. For example, Northern blot analysis will result in information on RNA size, the existence of splice variants, and closely related sequences. However, this type of assay is not sensitive or quantitative and requires a large amount of sample and large differences between treatments. Commonly used assays such as slot-blots and RNase protection are more quantitative and have improved sensitivity. Nonetheless, in terms of the amount of sample required, detection of small differences, and ability to examine many genes in a large number of samples, PCR stands above the more conventional procedures.

There are several terms that will be used in this chapter that are specific to quantitative RT–PCR, as outlined below. Also, many of the terms used are not universally accepted (i.e., internal standard versus external standard) and require more of a description. For detailed description of the terms, comparisons of the various PCR-based assays, and analysis of linearity, reproducibility, and validity, the reader is directed to several review articles.[3-9]

Definitions

Internal Standard (IS): A type of control molecule that can be used to minimize tube-to-tube variability in amplification efficiency. Normally an IS is a synthetic molecule that contains the same primer recognition sequences as the gene of interest. This type of amplification control is spiked into the PCR reaction.

External Standard (ES): A type of control that can be used to minimize differences in template (mRNA, cDNA, or DNA) concentration from sample-to-sample. Most often an ES is a housekeeping gene that is used in a coamplification type of quantitation. This control is not added to each sample, because it is present in a finite amount in each tube. Care must be taken to assure that the housekeeping gene is not affected by the treatment condition. Typical external standards include actin, tubulin, or glyceraldehyde 3-phosphate dehydrogenase.

Template: Any cDNA or DNA that contains primer recognition sites and can be PCR amplified.

Target gene: The target gene is the gene of interest and is a term used to differentiate from the internal standard, external standard, or artifact templates.

Linker gene: Specifically used to describe a template used to create a synthetic molecule in the synthesis of an internal standard.

Forward primer (FP): Analogous to the 5' or upstream primer (usp).

Reverse primer (RP): Same as the 3' or downstream primer (dsp).

Crossover point: In competitive RT–PCR, the concentration of internal standard where the PCR products for the target and the internal standard are equivalent.

II.   Construction of Internal Standards

The internal standard (IS) is a key reagent in the quantitation of template using PCR.[5] The requirement of an internal standard is necessitated by the fact that there is a large amount of tube-to-tube variability in amplification efficiency. For example, if 10 tubes of seemingly identical reagents are PCR amplified, there could be as much as a threefold difference in the amount of product formed. If an IS was coamplified with the target, the efficiency of amplification in each tube could be corrected and this threefold difference could easily be negated.

There is an infinite variety of methods that can be used to produce an internal standard. Four of the most popular are outlined in the pages that follow. One should keep in mind the requirements of their internal standard, i.e., what criteria are being applied to assess whether an IS is adequate. Some of the major criteria are listed below:

- **An internal standard should amplify with the same efficiency as the target**
  This is usually accomplished by incorporating the target gene's primer sequences

in the IS and making it of approximately the same length as the target PCR product.

- **The product from the IS must be easy to resolve from the target.** This may be accomplished by making the two products different enough in length to be resolved on a gel or by adding a restriction enzyme recognition site.
- **The internal standard should control for differences in reverse transcription efficiency.** This is easily accomplished by making the IS an RNA molecule with a poly(A)+ tail.

A. Recombinant RNA Synthesis

1. Basic Considerations

The method described below[10] for the synthesis of a recombinant RNA molecule is very similar to subcloning by PCR. In most PCR reactions, only the 3' end of the primer is required for efficient amplification. Therefore, extra sequences can be added to the 5' end of the molecule that will not be involved in the actual amplification. These extra sequences can be restriction enzyme recognition sites (i.e., in subcloning), primer or hybridization sites, poly(A)+ tails, or RNA polymerase sites. There is very little difference between PCR utilizing 18-mers and 40 to 60-mers except for the annealing temperature and possibly the annealing time. Also, generally the efficiency of amplification is lower with the long primers. Therefore, amplify multiple tubes or reamplify the primary products in order to obtain enough DNA for subsequent steps (see Figure 2.2).

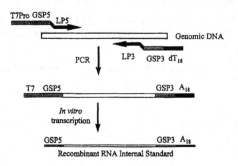

Figure 2.2
Construction of a synthetic RNA internal standard. The design of the internal standard primers are as follows (5' to 3'): *Forward Primer,* T7 promoter sequence (T7 Pro), gene-specific forward primer (GSP5), linker gene forward primer (LP5); *Reverse Primer,* 15 to 18 nucleotide dT tail (dT$_{18}$), gene-specific reverse primer (GSP3), linker gene reverse primer (LP3). Note that the spacer primer sequences are designed so that ANY sequence can be inserted. The key is to find a linker sequence that will ultimately result in a PCR product that is different from that of the target. The primers used in the making of the internal standard are quite long (around 60 bp), but only the 3' will anneal and amplify. The rest of the primer will be incorporated into the PCR product.

46   PCR Protocols in Molecular Toxicology

2.   Internal Standard Amplification

Protocol

1. Assemble the following in the order listed, enough for five reactions.

Component	Volume	Final Concentration
ddH$_2$O	162 µl	—
MgCl$_2$ (25 mM)	36	3 mM
10X PCR Buffer	30	1X
dATP (100 mM)	1.2	0.4 mM
dCTP (100 mM)	1.2	0.4 mM
dGTP (100 mM)	1.2	0.4 mM
dTTP (100 mM)	1.2	0.4 mM
Forward IS primer (10 pmol/µl)	18	0.6 nM
Reverse IS primer (10 pmol/µl)	18	0.6 nM

2. Place PCR mix at 85°C for at least 3 min. Meanwhile, pipet 5 µl genomic DNA (2 ng/µl, 10 ng total; source depends on species of linker primers) into each of five tubes.

3. Add 2 µl *Taq* DNA polymerase (5 U/µl) to the preheated PCR mix.

4. Briefly heat tubes containing genomic DNA to 85°C in a heat block or thermocycler. Add 45 µl PCR mix with *Taq* to each DNA sample. Cap and vortex samples.

5. Immediately amplify using the following cycle profile (Perkin Elmer 9600 or equivalent):

Denature	94°C 4 min
	<u>Cycle (30X)</u>
Denature	94°C 20 sec
Anneal	59°C 30 sec
Elongate	72°C 30 sec
Elongate	72°C 5 min
Store	4°C

Analysis of Gene Expression

6. Pool the multiple IS reactions and purify, using any procedure that will remove the unincorporated primers. This may be done using glass wool (i.e., Wizard Preps, Promega Corp., Madison, WI) or centrifugation (i.e., Microcon-100, Amicon Corp, Beverly, MA) following the manufacturer's suggestions.

7. Analyze 5μl on an agarose gel. (See Chapter 6). At this point you may not be able to see a PCR band, depending on the efficiency of the primers. If you cannot see a product, continue with Step 8. If a prominent band is observed, continue with *in vitro* transcription.

8. Dilute PCR products 1:100 with ddH$_2$O and amplify multiple tubes (5 to 6 tubes) as shown in Steps 1 through 5.

9. Pool and purify PCR products as stated in Step 6. Analyze PCR products on an agarose gel. If the product is not clean enough, gel purify the appropriate band (Chapter 6). If a discrete IS band is observed, continue with the *in vitro* transcription protocol as listed below.

3. In Vitro Transcription

Protocol

1. Prepare the following mix, in the order shown.

Component	Volume	Final Concentration
5X Transcription buffer	20 μl	1X
100 m*M* DTT	10 μl	10 m*M*
rRNasin (30 U/μl)	2.5 μl	75 U
rATP (10 m*M*)	5 μl	0.5 m*M*
rCTP (10 m*M*)	5 μl	0.5 m*M*
rGTP (10 m*M*)	5 μl	0.5 m*M*
rUTP (10 m*M*)	5 μl	0.5 m*M*
IS PCR product	45 μl	100 ng-1 μg
T7 RNA polymerase (15 to 20 U/μl)	2 μl	20 U

2. Incubate for 1 to 2 h at 37°C.

3. Add 2 μl RNase-free DNase (1 U/μl). Incubate for 15 to 30 min at 37°C.

4. Add 100 μl TE-buffered phenol. Vortex for 1 min and centrifuge at 12,000 × *g* for 10 min.

5. Transfer upper phase to a fresh tube. Add 100 μl chloroform/isoamyl alcohol (24:1). Vortex and centrifuge at 12,000 × *g* for 10 min.

6. Transfer upper phase to a fresh tube. Add 50 μl 10 *N* ammonium acetate (pH 4.0) and 500 μl ethanol. Precipitate at –20°C for 30 min.

7. Centrifuge at 12,000 × g for 10 min. Wash with 70% ethanol.
8. Quantitate RNA using absorbance at 260 nm. [Note: to quantitate RNA use the following formula: $ABS_{260} \times 0.04 \times$ dilution factor = µg/µl].
9. Calculate the molecules/µl of IS using the following formula:

$$\frac{\mu g/\mu l}{(330\,\mu g/\mu mol/bp \cdot bp\,IS)} \cdot 6.02 \times 10^{17}\ \text{mlcls/}\mu\text{mole}$$

The 330 × bp is an approximation for the molecular weight of the internal standard. For example, a 0.1 mg/ml solution of a 400 bp IS would be 4.56×10^{11} mlcls/µl.

10. Once an IS is produced, make serial dilutions in ddH$_2$O (i.e., 10^{10} mlcls/µl, 10^9 mlcls/µl, ...). Freeze the stock IS at –80°C in small aliquots to avoid repeated freezing and thawing. The diluted IS may be stored at –20°C for several weeks.
11. Proceed with testing of the IS as described in section II.E.

B. Low-Stringency Amplification

1. Basic Considerations

The basic theory behind this approach is that at low stringency a PCR product may be produced that has a different size than the target DNA (see Figure 2.3). The primer sequences are being incorporated even at the lower stringency,

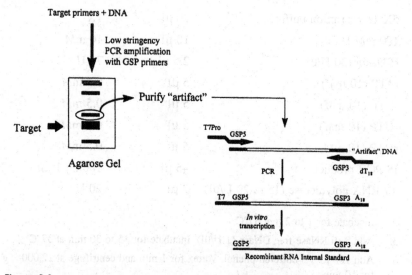

Figure 2.3
Low-stringency amplification to produce an internal standard. Genomic DNA is amplified under low stringency using the target primers (gene-specific primers, GSP5 and GSP3). Subsequently, a product that is sufficiently different from the target PCR product is purified. This artifactual product contains the GSP sites and may be used as a template for the incorporation of T7 and polyA sequences.

Analysis of Gene Expression

but the distance between them will be different than under stringent conditions. Therefore, this is an alternative to using a linker gene. The advantage of this approach is that shorter primers may be used and a wide range of sizes may be selected for the final internal standard. The initial steps are described below, while the final portions of the internal standard construction (*in vitro* transcription) are the same as described above.

2. Internal Standard Amplification

Protocol

1. Assemble the following in the order listed, enough for five reactions.

Component	Volume	Final Concentration
ddH$_2$O	162 µl	—
MgCl$_2$ (25 mM)	36	3 mM
10X PCR Buffer	30	1X
dATP (100 mM)	1.2	0.4 mM
dCTP (100 mM)	1.2	0.4 mM
dGTP (100 mM)	1.2	0.4 mM
dTTP (100 mM)	1.2	0.4 mM
Forward IS primer (10 pmol/µl)	18	0.6 nM
Reverse IS primer (10 pmol/µl)	18	0.6 nM

2. Place PCR mix at 85°C for at least 3 min. Meanwhile, pipet 5 µl genomic DNA (2 ng/µl, 10 ng total) into each of five tubes.
3. Add 2 µl *Taq* DNA polymerase (5 U/µl) to the preheated PCR mix.
4. Briefly heat tubes containing genomic DNA to 85°C in a heat block or thermocycler. Add 45 µl PCR mix with *Taq* to each DNA sample. Cap and vortex samples.
5. Immediately amplify using the following cycle profile (Perkin Elmer 9600 or equivalent):

Denature	94°C 4 min
	<u>CyCle (30X)</u>

Denature	94°C 20 sec
Anneal	42°C 30 sec

50   PCR Protocols in Molecular Toxicology

Elongate   72°C 30 sec

Elongate   72°C 5 min
Store   4°C

6. Pool the multiple IS reactions and purify using any procedure that will remove the unincorporated primers. This may be done using glass wool (i.e., Wizard Preps, Promega Corp., Madison, WI) or centrifugation (i.e., Microcon-100, Centricon) following the manufacturer's suggestions.

7. Add loading dye to the sample and resolve all of the PCR reaction on a low-melting agarose gel. (See Chapter 6). Run molecular weight markers on the same gel to determine the approximate size of the products. The most prominent band is usually the specific product.

Note: *It may be beneficial to run an aliquot of the specific PCR product (i.e., the product produced by the gene-specific primers) on the same gel for comparison.*

8. Identify a nonspecific product that differs by approximately 20%, if possible. This band may be larger or smaller than the specific product. Carefully excise this band and purify. (See Chapter 6).

9. Quantitate the amount of PCR product isolated and dilute to 10 ng/µl.

10. Continue with the synthesis of PCR product with a T7 RNA polymerase site as discussed above if an RNA molecule is desired.

Note: *An alternative to producing T7 RNA polymerase sites by PCR is to clone the PCR product into a plasmid that contains this motif (pCRII, Invitrogen Corp.; pTarget, Promega Corp). Cloning of PCR products is discussed in Chapter 6.*

C.   Amplification Across an Intron

1.   Basic Design

The construction of an internal standard by amplification across an intron is highly dependent on knowledge of the genomic sequence of the target gene. Two considerations must be made when utilizing this approach: 1) the intron must be small enough so that efficiency of amplification is not too dissimilar between internal standard and target; and 2) the exons must contain primer sequences that meet all the criteria stated previously to be acceptable, PLUS span an intron (see Figure 2.4). If you are fortunate enough to be interested in a gene that is amenable to this approach, it certainly is the easiest way to

Analysis of Gene Expression

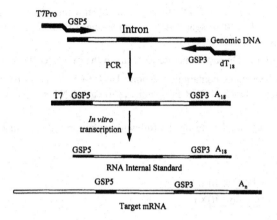

Figure 2.4
Amplification across an intron to produce an internal standard. Genomic DNA is used as a template, and primers are designed to amplify across a known intron. T7 and polyA sites may be included on the GSP primers for the production of rcRNA molecule. In this method of internal standard construction, the target mRNA PCR product will always be smaller.

make a suitable internal standard. Once again, the latter portions of the procedure, i.e., *in vitro* transcription, are covered elsewhere.

2. Internal Standard Amplification

Protocol

1. Assemble the following in the order listed, enough for five reactions.

Component	Volume	Final Concentration
ddH$_2$O	162 µl	—
MgCl$_2$ (25 mM)	36	3 mM
10X PCR Buffer	30	1X
dATP (100 mM)	1.2	0.4 mM
dCTP (100 mM)	1.2	0.4 mM
dGTP (100 mM)	1.2	0.4 mM
dTTP (100 mM)	1.2	0.4 mM
Forward IS primer (10 pmol/µl)	18	0.6 nM
Reverse IS primer (10 pmol/µl)	18	0.6 nM

PCR Protocols in Molecular Toxicology

2. Place PCR mix at 85°C for at least 3 min. Meanwhile, pipet 5 µl genomic DNA (2 ng/µl, 10 ng total; source depends on species of linker primers) into each of five tubes.

3. Add 2 µl *Taq* DNA polymerase (5 U/µl) to the preheated PCR mix.

4. Briefly heat tubes containing genomic DNA to 85°C in a heat block or thermocycler. Add 45 µl PCR mix with *Taq* to each DNA sample. Cap and vortex samples.

5. Immediately amplify using the following cycle profile (Perkin Elmer 9600 or equivalent):

Denature	94°C 4 min
	<u>Cycle (30X)</u>

Denature	94°C 20 sec
Anneal	59°C 30 sec
Elongate	72°C 30 sec

Elongate	72°C 5 min
Store	4°C

6. Pool the multiple IS reactions and purify using any procedure that will remove the unincorporated primers. This may be done using glass wool (i.e., Wizard Preps, Promega Corp., Madison, WI) or centrifugation (i.e., Microcon-100, Centricon), following the manufacturer's suggestions.

7. Analyze 5 µl on an agarose gel. (See Chapter 6). At this point you may not be able to see a PCR band, depending on the efficiency of the primers. If you cannot see a product, continue with Step 8. If a prominent band is observed continue with *in vitro* transcription.

8. Dilute PCR products 1:100 and amplify multiple tubes (5 to 6) as shown in Step 1.

9. Pool and purify PCR products as stated in Step 6. Analyze PCR products on an agarose gel. If the product is not clean enough, gel purify the appropriate band. If a discrete IS band is observed, continue with the *in vitro* transcription protocol as described above.

D. Internal Standard with a Mutated Restriction Enzyme Site

1. Basic Considerations

Having an internal standard that is only one base pair different than the target is the ideal situation. You are guaranteed identical primer annealing, little

Analysis of Gene Expression

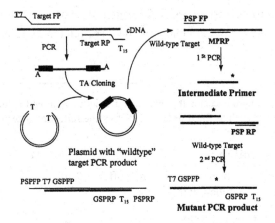

Figure 2.5
Construction of an internal standard using PCR mutagenesis. PCR amplification of the target gene cDNA is performed using gene-specific primers (GSP) that contain the T7 RNA polymerase recognition site and a polyT tail. After amplification, the wild-type, or normal, PCR product is ligated into a plasmid vector using a TA cloning method. This wild-type plasmid serves as a template for two successive rounds of PCR amplification. In the first PCR reaction, a mutant reverse primer (MPRP) and a plasmid-specific forward primer (PSPFP) are used to amplify the intermediate primer. The mutant reverse primer contains a single nucleotide difference compared with the wild-type sequence and may add or remove a unique restriction enzyme site. In the second round of PCR amplification, the intermediate primer and the plasmid-specific reverse primer (PSRP) are used to amplify the full-length, mutated PCR product. This product may be used in an *in vitro* transcription reaction to generate an RNA internal standard.

difference in secondary structure, and, since the lengths of the PCR products are the same, the overall amplification efficiency should be equivalent. The primary difficulty lies in the synthesis of this molecule. In addition, one must also assume that the restriction endonuclease being used is highly efficient.

There are three basic steps to constructing this internal standard: 1) cloning the target gene PCR product. The basic protocols for cloning PCR products will be discussed below and in Chapter 4 and utilize the fact that *Taq* DNA polymerase adds a single adenosine on the 3′ end of the PCR product; 2) a two-step method for site-directed mutagenesis using PCR.[11] The particular method to be discussed can be used to either remove or add a unique restriction endonuclease site; and 3) *in vitro* transcription of the mutated product resulting in a recombinant RNA molecule. The outline of methods is shown in Figure 2.5.

The design of the mutant reverse primer is a critical consideration. It must either remove or add a unique restriction enzyme site. Therefore, a map of all endonuclease sites in the target PCR product is warranted. An example is given below which will remove an Xba I site.[11]

XbaI site

```
5′    ATGAAAAAGTCACTGGAACTCTAGATAACGAGGGAACTG  3′  Target sequence
           3′ TGACCTTGAGCTCTATTGC  5′              Mutagenic primer
                            *
```

54 PCR Protocols in Molecular Toxicology

2. Construction of PCR Cloning Vector

For a review of the roles of cloning vectors, see references 12 and 13.

Protocol

1. Choose a plasmid vector that contains a unique, blunt-end cutting restriction enzyme site such as SmaI or EcoRV. Set up the following digestion reaction:

ddH$_2$O	up to 20 μl
10X restriction enzyme buffer (supplied with enzyme)	2 μl
Cloning vector	5 μg
Blunt-end cutting enzyme	10 units

2. Allow the digestion to proceed at 37°C for at least three hours. Heat inactivate the enzyme at 65°C for 15 min.
3. Add 20 μl (1 volume) TE-buffered phenol/chloroform (1:1, v/v), vortex for 1 min, and centrifuge for 2 min at 12,000 × g.
4. Carefully remove the top, aqueous layer and transfer to a fresh tube. Add 10 μl (0.5 volume) 7.5 M ammonium acetate and 40 μl (2 volumes) chilled 100% ethanol. Vortex briefly and precipitate at –70°C for 30 min.
5. Centrifuge at 12,000 × g for 10 min, decant the supernatant and briefly rinse the pellet with 1 ml 70% ethanol. Dry the pellet for 15 min under vacuum and dissolve the linearized plasmid in 15 μl ddH$_2$O.
6. Take 2 μl of the sample to measure the concentration of the DNA using UV spectroscopy. Estimate the amount of DNA present using the following formula:

$$\mu g/\mu l \text{ sample} = \text{Absorption at 260nm} \times 0.04 \ \mu g/\mu l \times \text{dilution factor}$$

7. Since circularized, uncut plasmid can cause very high background in subsequent experiments, care must be taken to assure that only the cut, linearized plasmid is present. Take a 2 μl aliquot and resolve on an 0.8% agarose gel. If complete digestion did not occur, repeat Steps 1 through 7.
8. This plasmid can now be used to generate a T-overhang vector. Set up the following reaction in the order listed, enough for five reactions:

Component	Volume	Final Concentration
ddH$_2$O	171 μl	—
MgCl$_2$ (25 mM)	40	3 mM
10X Buffer	25	1X

Analysis of Gene Expression

Component	Volume	Final Concentration
dTTP (100 mM)	1.2	0.4 mM
Linearized plasmid	10	up to 1 µg/tube
Taq DNA polymerase (5 U/µl)	2	2 units/tube

9. Pipet 50 µl into each of four tubes. Incubate at 72°C for 1 h. Pool the four reactions.

10. Add 200 µl (1 volume) TE-buffered phenol/chloroform (1:1, v/v), vortex for 1 min, and centrifuge for 2 min at 12,000 × *g*.

11. Carefully remove the top, aqueous layer and transfer to a fresh tube. Add 100 µl (0.5 volume) 7.5 M ammonium acetate and 400 µl (2 volumes) chilled 100% ethanol. Vortex briefly and precipitate at –70°C for 30 min.

12. Centrifuge at 12,000 × *g* for 10 minutes, decant the supernatant, and briefly rinse the pellet with 1 ml 70% ethanol. Dry the pellet for 15 min under vacuum and dissolve the linearized plasmid in 50 µl ddH$_2$O.

13. Take 2 µl of the sample to measure the concentration of the DNA using UV spectroscopy. Estimate the amount of DNA present using the following formula:

$$\mu g/\mu l \text{ sample} = \text{Absorption at 260 nm} \times 0.04\ \mu g/\mu l \times \text{dilution factor}$$

3. Generation of Wild-Type Plasmid

1. If the plasmid purified above does not contain T7 RNA polymerase and poly(A)+ sites, primers are designed with a T7 RNA polymerase recognition site and a poly T tail as discussed previously (see Section II.A). If the plasmid does have these sites, the target primers may be used.

2. Assemble the following in the order listed, enough for five reactions.

Component	Volume	Final Concentration
ddH$_2$O	162 µl	—
MgCl$_2$ (25 mM)	36	3 mM
10X PCR Buffer	30	1X
dATP (100 mM)	1.2	0.4 mM
dCTP (100 mM)	1.2	0.4 mM
dGTP (100 mM)	1.2	0.4 mM
dTTP (100 mM)	1.2	0.4 mM
Forward IS primer (10 pmol/µl)	18	0.6 nM
Reverse IS primer (10 pmol/µl)	18	0.6 nM

56 PCR Protocols in Molecular Toxicology

3. Place PCR mix 85°C for at least 3 min. Meanwhile, pipet 5 µl genomic DNA (2 ng/µl, 10 ng total; source depends on species of linker primers) or cDNA (100 ng/tube) into each of five tubes.

4. Add 2 µl *Taq* DNA polymerase (5 U/µl) to the preheated PCR mix.

5. Briefly heat tubes containing genomic DNA to 85°C in a heat block or thermocycler. Add 45 µl PCR mix with *Taq* to each DNA sample. Cap and vortex samples.

6. Immediately amplify using the following cycle profile (Perkin Elmer 9600 or equivalent):

Denature	94°C 4 min
	Cycle (30X)

Denature	94°C 20 sec
Anneal	59°C 30 sec
Elongate	72°C 30 sec

Elongate	72°C 5 min
Store	4°C

7. Pool the multiple IS reactions and purify using any procedure that will remove the unincorporated primers. This may be done using glass wool (i.e., Wizard Preps, Promega Corp., Madison, WI) or centrifugation (i.e., Microcon-100, Centricon), following the manufacturer's suggestions.

8. Analyze 5 µl on an agarose gel. (See Chapter 6). At this point you may not be able to see a PCR band, depending on the efficiency of the primers. If you cannot see a product, continue with Step 9. If a prominent band is observed continue with *in vitro* transcription.

9. Dilute PCR products 1:100 and amplify multiple tubes (5 to 6) as shown in Step 1.

10. Pool and purify PCR products as stated in Step 7. Analyze PCR products on an agarose gel. If the product is not clean enough, gel purify the appropriate band.

11. Set up the following ligation reactions, on ice:

Ligation Reaction

ddH$_2$O	up to 20 µl
10X Ligation buffer	2
Linearized plasmid	100 ng
PCR product	400 ng

Analysis of Gene Expression   57

T4 DNA ligase	10 units

Control Ligation Reaction

ddH$_2$O	up to 20 µl
10X Ligation buffer	2
Linearized plasmid	100 ng
PCR product	0
T4 DNA ligase	10 units

12. Incubate at 15°C overnight. Stop the reaction at 70°C for 10 min.

13. For heat-shock transformation of *E. coli* follow the procedures listed below. Each bacterial strain has different optimal transformation conditions. The appropriate conditions for DH5α cells (Gibco, BRL), a good, standard efficiency strain that allows for blue/white screening, are given.[13]

    i.   Thaw competent *E. coli* on ice.

    ii. Add 10 µl ligation reaction to 50 µl *E. coli* and let sit on ice for 30 min.

    iii. Place in 37°C water for 30 sec.

    iv. Put tubes back on ice for 2 min.

    v.   Add 1 mL LB or SOC media (See Chapter 6).

    vi. Shake tubes (220 rpm) at 37°C for 1 h.

    vii. Spin briefly in a microfuge, remove supernatant and *gently* resuspend in 100 µl LB media.

    viii. Spread 90 µl and 10 µl on each of two LB agar plates (with IPTG and X-Gal if blue/white screening is performed) containing the appropriate antibiotic.

    ix. Grow inverted at 37°C overnight

14. Check colonies for the presence of inserts as discussed in Chapter 4.

4. PCR Mutagenesis

Protocol

1. Assemble the following in the order listed, enough for five reactions. Note that the nucleotide concentration is at 100 µ*M*, which may prevent some random mutations from being incorporated.

Component	Volume	Final Concentration
ddH2O	162 µl	—
MgCl$_2$ (25 m*M*)	36	3 m*M*

10X PCR Buffer	30	1X
dATP (10 mM)	3	0.1 mM
dCTP (10 mM)	3	0.1 mM
dGTP (10 mM)	3	0.1 mM
dTTP (10 mM)	3	0.1 mM
Mutagenic primer (10 pmol/μl)	18	0.6 nM
Plasmid-specific FP (10 pmol/μl)	18	0.6 nM

2. Place PCR mix at 85°C for at least 3 min. Meanwhile, pipet 5 μl genomic wild-type plasmid DNA (1 ng/μl, 5 ng total) into each of five tubes.

3. Add 2 μl *Taq* DNA polymerase (5 U/μl) to the preheated PCR mix.

4. Briefly heat tubes containing genomic DNA to 85°C in a heat block or thermocycler. Add 45 μl PCR mix with *Taq* to each DNA sample. Cap and vortex samples.

5. Immediately amplify using the following cycle profile (Perkin Elmer 9600 or equivalent):

Denature	94°C 4 min
	<u>Cycle (30X)</u>
Denature	94°C 20 sec
Anneal	45°C 30 sec
Elongate	72°C 30 sec
Elongate	72°C 5 min
Store	4°C

6. Pool the multiple IS reactions and purify using any procedure that will remove the unincorporated primers. This may be done using glass wool (i.e., Wizard Preps, Promega Corp., Madison, WI) or centrifugation (i.e., Microcon-100, Centricon), following the manufacturer's suggestions.

7. Analyze 5 μl on an agarose gel. (See Chapter 6). Quantitate the amount of product formed by absorbance at 260 nm.

8. Assemble the second PCR reaction as follows in the order listed, enough for five reactions.

9. Place PCR mix at 85°C for at least 3 min. Meanwhile, pipet 5 μl genomic wild-type plasmid DNA (1 ng/μl, 5 ng total) into each of five tubes.

Analysis of Gene Expression

Component	Volume	Final Concentration
ddH₂O	162 μl	—
MgCl₂ (25 mM)	36	3 mM
10X PCR Buffer	30	1X
dATP (100 mM)	0.6	0.2 mM
dCTP (100 mM)	0.6	0.2 mM
dGTP (100 mM)	0.6	0.2 mM
dTTP (100 mM)	0.6	0.2 mM
Plasmid-specific RP (10 pmol/μl)	18	0.6 nM
Intermediate product (10 pmol/μl)	18	0.6 nM

10. Add 2 μl *Taq* DNA polymerase (5 U/μl) to the preheated PCR mix.

11. Briefly heat tubes containing genomic DNA to 85°C in a heat block or thermocycler. Add 45 μl PCR mix with *Taq* to each DNA sample. Cap and vortex samples.

12. Immediately amplify using the following cycle profile (Perkin Elmer 9600 or equivalent):

Denature	94°C 4 min
	<u>Cycle (30X)</u>
Denature	94°C 20 sec
Anneal	60°C 30 sec
Elongate	72°C 30 sec
Elongate	72°C 5 min
Store	4°C

13. Pool and gel purify the PCR reaction to remove the intermediate primer. Procedures for gel purification are given in Chapter 6.

14. Chloroform/phenol extract the PCR product as discussed above.

15. Proceed with *in vitro* transcription as described in Section II.A.3.

60   PCR Protocols in Molecular Toxicology

E.   Testing Internal Standards

1.   Basic Considerations

As mentioned previously, in order for the rcRNA to be useful in quantitative RT–PCR, it must amplify with roughly the same efficiency as the target mRNA, give a single PCR product, and be easily resolved from the target. Before continuing with quantitation, it is advisable to perform two simple studies to evaluate the internal standard you synthesized. The first is to amplify a dilution series of the rcRNA with or without an RNA sample. This will be useful in subsequent range-finding assays and will also determine whether the rcRNA results in a single product that is easily separated from the target. The second study is to roughly gauge the efficiency of your internal standard as compared to the target. This is most often examined by removing PCR products at various times in the PCR reaction. Both types of evaluation are discussed below.

2.   Amplification of a Dilution Series of rcRNA (Standard RT–PCR Procedures)

Protocol

1. Dilute the internal standard to 10^{11} molecules/2 µl. From this stock, make a series of 1:10 dilutions in ddH_2O (i.e., 20 µl 10^{11}/2 µl + 180 µl ddH_2O). To test the sensitivity of the primers, proceed to 10^3 molecules/2 µl.

Note: *Internal standards are small molecules that can easily become air-borne and contaminate future experiments. Whenever possible, utilize aerosol barrier tips and work in a well-ventilated area. Be very careful when handling rcRNA and always keep on ice to prevent degradation. The diluted rcRNA may be stored at $-20°C$, while the stock solutions should be maintained at $-80°C$ in small aliquots to prevent frequent freeze–thaw cycles.*

2. Prepare the following for the first-strand cDNA synthesis and place on ice. The recipe is enough for eight tubes. (The final reaction volume will be 20 µl).

Component	*µl*	*Final Concentration*
ddH_2O	95	—
$MgCl_2$ (25 mM)	36	5 mM
10X PCR Buffer	18	1X
dATP (100 mM)	1.8	1 mM

Analysis of Gene Expression

dCTP (100 mM)	1.8	1 mM
dGTP (100 mM)	1.8	1 mM
dTTP (100 mM)	1.8	1 mM
Oligo(dT)$_{15}$ (0.5 mg/ml)*	2.3	6 µg/ml
rRNasin (30 U/µl)	2.3	7.5 U

*Random hexamers may be substituted for Oligo(dT)$_{15}$

3. On ice, add 2 µl of serially diluted IS per PCR tube (10^9 to 10^3 mlcls/2 µl) plus one tube of 2 µl ddH$_2$O.

4. Add 2.5 µl (500 U) MMLV reverse transcriptase to the cDNA mixture. Vortex.

Note: *MMLV is the most common type of reverse transcriptase used in cDNA synthesis. AMV reverse transcriptase may be substituted, but use 5 units/tube.*

5. Add 18 µl cDNA mix to the PCR tubes containing internal standard. Cap tubes and vortex briefly to mix.

6. Place in the thermocycler and run the following program:

42°C for 15 min
95°C for 5 min
Store at 4°C

7. While the cDNA synthesis is proceeding, assemble the PCR mixture as follows, at room temperature.

Component	µl	*Final concentration (in PCR reaction)**
ddH$_2$O**	200	—
MgCl$_2$ (25 mM)**	36	4 mM
10X PCR Buffer	27	1X
Forward primer (10 pmol/µl)	5.4	6 pmol
Reverse primer (10 pmol/µl)	5.4	6 pmol

*   The cDNA reaction contains nucleotides, additional MgCl$_2$, and 10X buffer. The final concentration of nucleotides in the PCR is 400 µM.

** Must be optimized for each primer pair. The example given (4 mM MgCl$_2$) is adequate for most PCR reactions.

62 PCR Protocols in Molecular Toxicology

8. When cDNA reaction is complete, choose one of two methods for assembling the PCR reaction: hot start (Steps 9 through 12) or cold start (Steps 13 through 15).

Note: *Two different methods can be used in an attempt to decrease mis-priming and primer artifacts and to assure that all the tubes will start amplification simultaneously. In a hot start all the reagents (cDNA reactions, PCR master mix) are brought to 85°C prior to the addition of Taq. This will prevent the primers from binding to each other and will also dissociate the primers from the template. The easiest way to perform a hot start is to use a heat block that will hold the standard PCR tube. In a cold start the cDNA and the PCR mix are placed on ice. This method is technically easier and there is less chance of contamination, but the efficiency of amplification is much less than when using a hot start.*

Hot Start

9. Immediately prior to completion of the cDNA reaction, place the mix prepared in Step 7 in an 85°C heat block (3 to 5 minutes).

10. At the completion of the cDNA reaction, remove the tubes from the thermocycler and place them in an 85°C heat block. (The thermocycler may also be used as a surrogate heat block). Add 2.5 µl *Taq* DNA polymerase (5 U/µl) to the preheated mix. Vortex and return to the heat block.

11. Add 30 µl PCR mix directly to the tube containing the cDNA reaction in the heat block. Work quickly to avoid evaporation.

12. Place the reactions in the thermocycler only when it has reached at least 85°C. A sample PCR reaction is given below. The temperature, times, and cycles must be optimized for each primer pair.

Denature	94°C 4 min
	<u>Cycle (30X)</u>
Denature	94°C 20 sec
Anneal	55°C 30 sec
Elongate	72°C 30 sec
Elongate	72°C 5 min
Store	4°C

Cold Start

13. Prepare the PCR mix as suggested in Step 7. Place on ice.

Analysis of Gene Expression

14. At the completion of the cDNA reaction, remove the tubes from the thermocycler and place them on ice. Add 2.5 μl *Taq* DNA polymerase (5 U/μl) to the cold mix. Vortex and place back on ice

15. Add 30 μl PCR mix directly to the tube containing the cDNA reaction on ice.

16. Place the reactions in the thermocycler and run the optimized PCR program.

3. Amplification Efficiency of Internal Standard as Compared to the Target

The most accurate way to determine if your internal standard is amplifying with the same efficiency as the target is to examine the amount of product formed at various cycles. In addition, this cycle-based approach will verify that at the concentrations of IS and mRNA used, a plateau in product yield has not been reached. Usually, these types of studies require the use of a radioactive primer so that low cycle numbers can be examined. For a detailed description of how to assess amplification efficiency, see Section IV.

III. Competitive Quantitative RT–PCR

As mentioned previously, inherent in the polymerase chain reaction is a large amount of tube-to-tube variability in amplification efficiency. Any internal standard that meets the criteria discussed above can be used to reduce the concern of unequal rates of product formation in seemingly identical reactions. Once an IS is produced or obtained, the investigator has several options as to which method to use. Two similar competitive techniques (standard competitive RT–PCR and competitive RT–PCR with standard curve) and one kinetic, cycle-based approach will be discussed. There are several advantages of the competitive approach (See Table 2.1), and it is amenable to the majority of genes of interest. However, in rare instances the cycle-based approach is more desirable. This is especially true if the IS and the target have widely disparate amplification efficiencies.

TABLE 2.1

Advantages of Competitive vs. a Cycle-Based RT–PCR Approach

Competitive RT–PCR		Cycle-Based RT–PCR
✔	Nonradioactive and utilizes common laboratory equipment	
✔	Does not require pausing the thermocycler to remove sample or aliquots	
✔	Simple math and calculations	✔
✔	Relatively rapid and able to examine many samples	
	Can be used when IS and target have different amplification efficiencies	✔

A. General Competitive RT–PCR

1. Basic Considerations

The standard competitive RT–PCR approach is shown in Figure 2.6. The basis for this method is that the more competitor (i.e., IS) present, the less likely it is that the primers and *Taq* will be able to recognize and bind to the target cDNA and amplify. Therefore, despite the fact that all reagents are there in

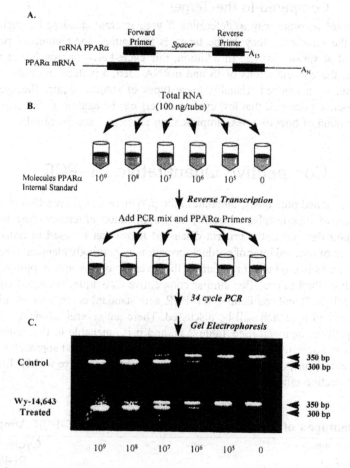

Figure 2.6
Basic competitive RT–PCR. The gene being examined is rat PPARα mRNA, to which an internal standard has been constructed, as depicted in Panel A. In basic competitive RT–PCR, a constant amount of RNA is used and a dilution series of IS is spiked into each tube (10^9 to 10^5 molecules/tube) as shown in Panel B. A representative ethidium bromide-stained agarose gel is shown in Panel C. Note that, as the amount of IS is increased (300 bp product), the intensity of the target product (350 bp) decreases. Also, the equivalency, or crossover, point is higher in the chemically treated samples (Wy 14,643, 10^7 molecules) than control (10^6 molecules), indicative of induction of PPARα mRNA. (Adapted from Sterchele, P. F., Sun, H., Peterson, R. E., and Vanden Heuvel, J. P., *Arch. Biochem. Biophys.*, 326, 281, 1996.)

Analysis of Gene Expression

extreme excess (i.e., primers, enzyme, $MgCl_2$, nucleotides) the reaction appears to be competitive.[5] That is, as the amount of competitor is increased, less and less target product is formed until eventually only the IS product is observed. When a dilution series of IS is spiked into a constant amount of RNA, it is possible to estimate the amount of a specific product present in the sample, as will be discussed subsequently.

2. Constant Amount of RNA with Serial Dilutions of Internal Standard

Protocol

Note: *The dilution range of IS to use is dependent on the expression level of the gene and how inducible it is by your treatment. The example given below can be used to determine relative amounts of a target gene in a sample and to compare treatments for a gene that is highly inducible. To detect small differences in expression between two samples, a narrower IS range is required. A relative amount of expression must first be determined (i.e., slightly greater than 10^6 molecules target per 100 ng total RNA), followed by utilizing a linear range of IS (2×10^7, 10^7, 8×10^6, 6×10^6, 4×10^6, 2×10^6, 10^6, 8×10^5).*

1. Dilute the internal standard to 10^{10} molecules/2 µl. From this stock, make a series of 1:10 dilutions in ddH_2O (i.e., 20 µl 10^{11}/2 µl + 180 µl ddH_2O). Proceed to 10^3 molecules/2 µl.

Note: *Internal standards are small molecules that can easily become airborne and contaminate future experiments. Whenever possible utilize aerosol barrier pipet tips and work in a well-ventilated area. Be very careful when handling rcRNA and always keep on ice to prevent degradation. The diluted rcRNA may be stored at $-20°C$, while the stock solutions should be maintained at $-80°C$, in aliquots if necessary to prevent frequent freeze–thaw cycles.*

2. Prepare the following for the first-strand cDNA synthesis and place on ice. The recipe is enough for eight tubes. (The final reaction volume will be 20 µl.) The RNA sample may be added directly to this mix to avoid pipetting error from tube to tube.

Component	µl	Final Concentration
ddH_2O	95	—
$MgCl_2$ (25 mM)	36	5 mM

10X PCR Buffer	18	1X
dATP (100 mM)	1.8	1 mM
dCTP (100 mM)	1.8	1 mM
dGTP (100 mM)	1.8	1 mM
dTTP (100 mM)	1.8	1 mM
Oligo(dT)$_{15}$ (0.5 mg/ml)*	2.3	6 µg/ml
rRNasin (30 U/µl)	2.3	7.5 U
Total RNA sample (0.05 µg/µl)	16	100 ng/tube

* Random hexamers may be substituted for Oligo(dT)$_{15}$.

3. On ice, add 2 µl of serially diluted IS per PCR tube (10^9 to 10^2 mlcls/2 µl).

4. Add 2.5 µl (500 U) MMLV reverse transcriptase to the cDNA mixture. Vortex.

Note: *MMLV is the most common reverse transcriptase used in cDNA synthesis. AMV reverse transcriptase may be substituted, but use 5 units/tube.*

5. Add 18 µl cDNA mix to the PCR tubes containing internal standard. Cap tubes and vortex briefly to mix.

6. Place in the thermocycler and run the following program:

42°C for 15 min
95°C for 5 min
Store at 4°C

7. While the cDNA synthesis is proceeding, assemble the PCR mixture as follows, at room temperature:

Component	µ*l*	*Final concentration (in PCR reaction)**
ddH$_2$O**	200	—
MgCl$_2$ (25 mM)**	36	4 mM
10X PCR Buffer	27	1X

Analysis of Gene Expression

Forward primer (10 pmol/µl)	5.4	6 pmol
Reverse primer (10 pmol/µl)	5.4	6 pmol

* The cDNA reaction contains nucleotides, additional $MgCl_2$, and 10X buffer. The final concentration of nucleotides in the PCR is 400 µM.

** Must be optimized for each primer pair. The example given (4 mM $MgCl_2$) is adequate for most PCR reactions.

8. When the cDNA reaction is complete, choose one of two methods for assembly of the PCR reaction: hot start (Steps 9 through 12) or cold start (Steps 13 through 15).

Note: *Two different methods can be used in an attempt to decrease mispriming and primer artifacts and to assure that all the tubes will start amplification simultaneously. In a hot start, all the reagents (cDNA reactions, PCR master mix) are brought to 85°C prior to the addition of Taq. This will prevent the primers from binding to each other and will also dissociate the primers from the template. The easiest way to perform a hot start is to use a heat block that will hold the standard PCR tube. In a cold start the cDNA and the PCR mix are placed on ice. This method is technically easier, and there is less chance of contamination, but the efficiency of amplification is much less than when using a hot start.*

Hot Start

9. Immediately prior to completion of the cDNA reaction, place the mix prepared in Step 7 in an 85°C heat block (3 to 5 minutes).

10. At the completion of the cDNA reaction, remove the tubes from the thermocycler and place them in an 85°C heat block. (The thermocycler may also be used as a surrogate heat block). Add 2.5 µl *Taq* DNA polymerase (5 U/µl) to the preheated mix. Vortex and return to the heat block.

11. Add 30 µl PCR mix directly to the tube containing the cDNA reaction in the heat block. Work quickly to avoid evaporation.

12. Place the reactions in the thermocycler only when it has reached at least 85°C. A sample PCR reaction is given below. The temperature, times, and cycles must be optimized for each primer pair.

Denature	94°C 4 min
	<u>Cycle (30X)</u>
Denature	94°C 20 sec
Anneal	55°C 30 sec
Elongate	72°C 30 sec
Elongate	72°C 5 min
Store	4°C

Cold Start

13. Prepare the PCR mix as suggested in Step 7. Place on ice.
14. At the completion of the cDNA reaction, remove the tubes from the thermocycler and place them on ice. Add 2.5 µl *Taq* DNA polymerase (5 U/µl) to the cold mix. Vortex and place back on ice.
15. Add 30 µl PCR mix directly to the tube containing the cDNA reaction, on ice.
16. Place the reactions in the thermocycler and run the optimized PCR program.

3.   Quantitation

1. Add loading dye directly to each sample and resolve PCR products as discussed in Chapter 6.

Note: The method by which the PCR products are quantitated is highly dependent on the materials available. The example given below requires photographic equipment plus a scanning densitometer to quantitate the intensity of the bands. If the densitometer cannot scan the positive image (reflectance), a photographic negative may be scanned using materials common to autoradiography. In addition, there is also photographic equipment that can send a digitized image directly to a computer for analysis without the need for a photograph. This section will stress what to do after the PCR products have been analyzed.

2. Take a photograph of the ethidium bromide-stained gel.
3. Using a densitometer, find either volumes or peak heights of the target and IS PCR products and subtract background (i.e., density in a lane without any sample added).
4. Plot [volume IS/volume RNA] vs. molecules IS as shown in Figure 2.7. Use linear regression to draw a line through the data. (Note: often a data point is not

Analysis of Gene Expression

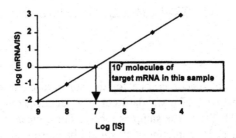

Figure 2.7
Hypothetical quantitation of amount of target mRNA present in a sample using standard competitive RT–PCR. The density of IS and target PCR products are determined and a ratio calculated (mRNA/IS). The log of mRNA/IS is plotted versus the log of the amount of IS spiked into each tube. The crossover or equivalency point is where the density of the target PCR product is equal to that of the IS (mRNA/IS = 1 or log(mRNA/IS) = 0). Linear regression may be used to approximate a line through the data.

in the linear region of the curve. If a point needs to be removed, it is usually the highest or lowest IS sample.)

5. The amount of target mRNA is determined by calculating the IS concentration where there is equivalent volume of IS to RNA (IS/RNA = 1, the crossover point). Calculate the molecules of target mRNA using the formula x = (1 − $y_{intercept}$)/slope, where x = the amount of target mRNA in your sample.

B. Quantitation Using a Standard Curve

1. Basic Considerations

This method is derived from general competitive RT–PCR but has been adapted to examine many samples concurrently.[15] For each experiment, one dilution series of IS is performed identically to the procedure described above. However, if you know the approximate level of expression of your target gene (i.e., 10^7 molecules/0.1 µg), many samples may be examined using this amount of IS spiked into the reaction. Range-finding experiments must be performed to determine an appropriate concentration of IS; that is, a concentration of IS is used that will result in strong band intensity for both the target mRNA and the IS. Subsequently, the ratio of band intensity for the IS versus RNA may be compared to the standard curve and expression levels estimated. Using this approach of quantitative RT–PCR, hundreds of samples may be examined in a single day, and the expenditure of resources will be limited. One limitation of utilizing one IS concentration for a series of tubes is that the expression levels for your target gene must be within three orders of magnitude across treatments.

This procedure has proven to be very efficient at examining dose–response relationships for various toxicant inducible genes[1,2,14,16,17] and is the preferred method of mRNA analysis performed by our laboratory.

2. Competitive RT–PCR with Standard Curve

Protocol

Set up two series of reactions, one for the standard curve and one for the samples to be analyzed. The standard curve is identical to that stated above for competitive RT–PCR. The samples receive one concentration of IS based on previous studies. This amount of IS should be close to the crossover point for the majority of samples.

1. Dilute the internal standard to 10^{10} molecules/2 µl. From this stock, make a series of 1:10 dilutions in ddH$_2$O (i.e., 20 µl 10^{11}/2 µl + 180 µl ddH$_2$O). Proceed to 10^3 molecules/2 µl.

Note: *Internal standards are small molecules that can easily become airborne and contaminate future experiments. Whenever possible, utilize aerosol barrier tips and work in a well-ventilated area. Be very careful when handling rcRNA and always keep it on ice to prevent degradation. The diluted rcRNA may be stored at –20°C, while the stock solutions should be maintained at –80°C, in aliquots if necessary, to prevent frequent freeze–thaw cycles.*

Mix A: Standard curve

2. Prepare the following for the first-strand cDNA synthesis and place on ice. The recipe is enough for eight tubes. (The final reaction volume will be 20 µl). The RNA sample may be added directly to this mix to avoid pipetting error from tube to tube.

Component	µl	Final Concentration
ddH$_2$O	95	—
MgCl$_2$ (25 mM)	36	5 mM
10X PCR Buffer	18	1X
dATP (100 mM)	1.8	1 mM
dCTP (100 mM)	1.8	1 mM
dGTP (100 mM)	1.8	1 mM
dTTP (100 mM)	1.8	1 mM
Oligo(dT)$_{15}$ (0.5 mg/ml)*	2.3	6 µg/ml

Analysis of Gene Expression

rRNasin (30 U/μl)	2.3	7.5 U
Total RNA sample (0.05 μg/μl)	16	100 ng/tube

* Random hexamers may be substituted for Oligo(dT)$_{15}$

Mix B: For the samples to be analyzed

Use the following worksheet to prepare the mix. Multiply the 1X volumes by the number of samples to be examined.

Component	Final Concentration	1X	nX
ddH$_2$O	—	10.5	
MgCl$_2$ (25 mM)	5 mM	4	
10X PCR Buffer	1X	2	
dATP (100 mM)	1 mM	0.2	
dCTP (100 mM)	1 mM	0.2	
dGTP (100 mM)	1 mM	0.2	
dTTP (100 mM)	1 mM	0.2	
Oligo(dT)$_{15}$ (0.5 mg/ml)*	6 μg/ml	0.25	
rRNasin (30 U/μl)	7.5 U	0.25	
Internal standard**	?	2	

  * Random hexamers may be substituted for Oligo(dT)$_{15}$.

** This must be determined from previous studies. Use an IS concentration that is close to the crossover point.

3. On ice, add 2 μl of serially diluted IS per PCR tube (10^9 to 10^2 mlcls/2 μl). Also on ice, add 2 μl RNA samples (diluted to 50 ng/μl) into separate PCR tubes.

4. Add 2.5 μl (500 U) MMLV reverse transcriptase to Mix A (standard curve). Vortex.

5. Add the equivalent of 0.3 μl per tube of MMLV reverse transcriptase to Mix B (samples). That is, if there are 25 samples to be examined, add 7.5 μl reverse transcriptase to Mix B.

6. On ice, add 18 μl cDNA Mix A to the PCR tubes containing internal standard and 18 μl cDNA Mix B to the PCR tubes containing the samples.

7. Place in the thermocycler and run the following program

42°C for 15 min
95°C for 5 min
Store at 4°C

PCR Protocols in Molecular Toxicology

8. While the cDNA synthesis is proceeding, assemble the PCR mixture as follows, at room temperature. The PCR mix is the same for the standard curve and the samples.

Component	Final concentration (in PCR reaction)*	1X	nX
ddH$_2$O**	—		22
MgCl$_2$ (25 mM)**	4 mM		4
10X PCR Buffer	1X		3
Forward primer (10 pmol/μl)	6 pmol		0.6
Reverse primer (10 pmol/μl)	6 pmol		0.6

* The cDNA reaction contains nucleotides, additional MgCl$_2$, and 10X buffer. The final concentration of nucleotides is 400 μM.

** Must be optimized for each primer pair. The example given (4 mM MgCl$_2$) is adequate for most PCR reactions.

9. When the cDNA reaction is complete, choose one of two methods for assembly of the PCR reaction: hot start (Steps 10 through 13) or cold start (Steps 14 through 16).

Note: *Two different methods can be used in an attempt to decrease mispriming and primer artifacts and to assure that all the tubes will start amplification simultaneously. In a hot start, all the reagents (cDNA reactions, PCR master mix) are brought to 85°C prior to the addition of Taq. This will prevent the primers from binding to each other and will also dissociate the primers from the template. The easiest way to perform a hot start is to use a heat block that will hold the standard PCR tube. In a cold start the cDNA and the PCR mix are placed on ice. This method is technically easier, and there is less chance of contamination, but the efficiency of amplification is much less than when using a hot start.*

Hot Start

10. Immediately prior to completion of the cDNA reaction, place the mix prepared in Step 8 in an 85°C heat block (3 to 5 minutes).

11. At the completion of the cDNA reaction, remove the tubes from the thermocycler and place them in an 85°C heat block. (The thermocycler may also be used as a surrogate heat block.) Add the equivalent of 0.25 μl per tube of *Taq* DNA polymerase (5 U/μl) to the preheated mix. Vortex and return to the heat block.

Analysis of Gene Expression

12. Add 30 µl PCR mix directly to the tube containing the cDNA reaction, in the heat block. Work quickly to avoid evaporation.
13. Place the reactions in the thermocycler only when it has reached at least 85°C. A sample PCR reaction is given below. The temperature, times, and cycles must be optimized for each primer pair.

Denature	94°C 4 min
	Cycle (30X)
Denature	94°C 20 sec
Anneal	55°C 30 sec
Elongate	72°C 30 sec
Elongate	72°C 5 min
Store	4°C

Cold Start

14. Prepare the PCR mix as suggested in Step 8. Place on ice.
15. At the completion of the cDNA reaction, remove the tubes from the thermocycler and place them on ice. Add the equivalent of 0.25 µl per tube of *Taq* DNA polymerase (5 U/µl) to the cold mix. Vortex and place back on ice.
16. Add 30 µl PCR mix directly to the tube containing the cDNA reaction, on ice.
17. Place the reactions in the thermocycler and run the optimized PCR program.

3. Quantitation

1. Add loading dye directly to each sample and resolve PCR products as discussed in Chapter 6.
2. Quantitate the intensity of the IS and target PCR products as discussed above.

Note: *The calculation of target mRNA using the standard curve requires various calculations and manipulations. In the following "Worksheet Template" an example is given to demonstrate how to use a computer spreadsheet to simplify the calculations. The first step is to calculate the amount of target mRNA in the standard sample, using methods identical to those stated above for competitive PCR. Next this standard curve is transformed so that direct determination of target mRNA can be ascertained based on the ratio of target to IS PCR products.*

Worksheet Template

1. Calculate log IS and log (mRNA/IS).

Arbitrary Absorbance Units

(IS)	log IS	mRNA	IS	Ratio (mRNA/IS)	log (mRNA/IS)
10^9	9	0.02	2.10	0.01	−2.0
10^8	9	0.08	1.50	0.12	−0.92
10^7	8	0.10	1.20	0.83	−0.081
10^6	7	0.98	0.80	1.22	0.086
10^5	6	1.58	0.16	9.88	0.99
10^4	5	2.12	0.02	101	2.0

2. Plot log (mRNA/IS) versus log (IS). Find slope and y-intercept and describe the data using linear regression (see Figure 2.8).

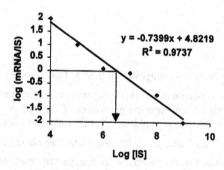

Figure 2.8
Example of linear regression analysis of PCR products.

        Slope = −0.748   y intercept = 4.82
        log (mRNA/IS) = −0.748(log[IS]) + 4.82
        Solve for log[IS] where intensity of the PCR product for mRNA equals that of IS:
            (mRNA/IS=1, log (mRNA/IS) = 0)
            0 = −0.748(log[IS]) + 4.82
            log[IS] = −6.52
            [IS]= 3.31 × 10^6 molecules

Therefore, there is 3.31 × 10^6 molecules target mRNA in this sample of mRNA.

3. Transform these data into a form that can be used for other samples. Use the amount of target mRNA to calculate a new ratio based on actual concentrations. Remember that the same amount of total mRNA was spiked into each tube.

Analysis of Gene Expression

		Concentration		Absorbance
		Ratio	log	log
(IS)	(mRNA)	(mRNA/IS)	(mRNA/IS)	(mRNA/IS)
10^9	3.31×10^6	0.003	−2.48	−2.0
10^8	3.31×10^6	0.03	−1.48	−0.92
10^7	3.31×10^6	0.03	−0.48	−0.81
10^6	3.31×10^6	0.30	0.48	0.086
10^5	3.31×10^6	3.02	1.48	0.99
10^4	3.31×10^6	30.2	2.48	2.0
			x-axis	y-axis

4. Plot absorbance unit ratio (mRNA/IS) versus concentration ratio (mRNA/IS) and use linear regression to describe the relationship (see Figure 2.9).

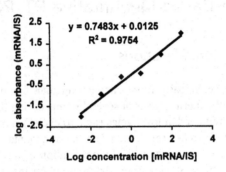

Figure 2.9
Transformed standard curve.

$$\text{slope} = 0.74 \qquad \text{y-intercept} = 0.01$$

In general terms the following equation can be used to calculate the amount of target gene in your sample. The derivation of this equation follows.

Let X = amount of target mRNA
D = (absorbance mRNA/ absorbance IS)
A = (amount of mRNA/amount of IS)
m = slope from above
b = y-intercept

Amount of target mRNA (X) = Amount of IS $\times 10^{(\log D - b)/m}$

$$\log(D) = m(\log(A)) + b$$
$$\frac{(\log(D) - b)}{m} = \log(A)$$
$$10^{(\log(D) - b)/m} = A, \text{ where A= amount of mRNA/ amount of IS}$$

5. Use this mathematical equation to calculate the amount of target mRNA in each of your samples. Five examples are given below, assuming that 10^6 molecule of internal standard was spiked into each sample.

Col(1) A.A.U. mRNA	Col(2) A.A.U. IS	Col(3) D mRNA/IS	Col(4) log(D)	Col(5) log(D) -b/m	Col(6) 10^{10} (col5)	Col(7) IS added	Col(8) Amt. target col(6) × col(7)
1.03	0.33	3.12	0.49	0.65	4.441105	1.00E+06	4.44E+06
0.45	0.65	0.69	−0.16	−0.23	0.593099	1.00E+06	5.93E+05
0.09	1.33	0.07	−1.17	−1.58	0.026484	1.00E+06	2.65E+04

IV. Cycle-Based Quantitative RT–PCR

A. Basic Considerations

This procedure is technically more challenging than competitive RT–PCR, requiring pausing the thermocycler at several points during the reaction. Also, since samples are removed at low cycles (i.e., 20 cycles), a radioactive primer is usually added to increase sensitivity. The major advantage of using cycle-based methods is that the efficiency of amplification of the internal standard and target are determined. Therefore, the assumption that the IS and target have equal amplification efficiency is negated. This method is particularly useful when comparing two products that are quite different in size or have different secondary structure (i.e., high G-C content).

Theoretically, PCR amplification results in a doubling of product with each cycle. In practice, the efficiency is less than 100% and the amount of product produced can be given by the formula:[3,4]

$$\text{Amount of final product } (Y) = A(1 + R)^n$$

where A is the initial amount of material (IS or target), R is the efficiency of amplification ($0 > R > 1$), and n is the number of cycles. It is possible to determine Y by measuring the extent of the ^{32}P-labeled primer incorporated. The efficiency can be deduced by a plot of $\log(Y) = \log(A) + n\log(1 + R)$, where the slope is equal to $\log(1 + R)$ (see Figure 2.10).

Either an IS or an external standard (ES) may be used in these methods. However, as discussed later, the use of four primers in one PCR may be troublesome. Also, when using an external standard, one can calculate A and compare samples to each other, but the values obtained will be relative (i.e., twofold induction). By using an internal standard, quantitative data may be

Analysis of Gene Expression

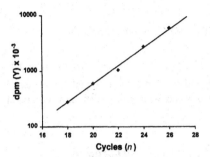

Figure 2.10
Yield (Y) versus cycle number (n). The efficiency of the PCR reaction can be deduced by a plot of $\log(Y) = \log(A) + n\log(1 + R)$, where the slope is equal to $\log(1 + R)$. A is the initial amount of material (IS or target), R is the efficiency of amplification ($0 > R > 1$), and n is the number of cycles.

obtained (i.e., 10^3 molecules per cell) and tube-to-tube variability is obviated. In this section, we will concentrate on the internal standard approach.

If the amplification of the internal standard (S) can be described as $Y_S = A_S(1 + R_S)^n$ and that of the target (T) with $Y_T = A_T(1 + R_T)^n$ the equations can be combined into

$$Y_T/Y_S = (A_T/A_S)[(1 + R_T)/(1 + R_S)]^n$$

Therefore:

$$\log(Y_T/Y_S) = \log(A_T/A_S) + n\log[(1 + R_T)/(1 + R_S)]$$

In a graph of $\log(Y_T/Y_S)$ versus n, the slope will be equal to $\log[(1 + R_T)/(1 + R_S)]$ and the y intercept equal to $\log(A_T/A_S)$. Therefore, if PCR analysis is done by varying the cycle number, and the Y_T and Y_S are measured, the ratio of A_T/A_S can be calculated from the y-intercept. Because we know the amount of internal standard spiked into each tube (A_S), the starting amount of target mRNA molecules can be determined (A_T).

B. Protocol

1. 5' Labeling of PCR Primer

Since tubes will be removed at early cycles, sensitivity is of paramount importance. Therefore, one or both of the primers may be labeled with (α-^{32}P-ATP as follows:

1. In a total volume of 10 µl, add the following on ice:
   - Forward or reverse PCR primer (100 pmol/µl)   1 µl
   - 10X forward exchange buffer   1 µl

- T4 polynucleotide kinase (10 U/μl)   1 μl
- [α-^{32}P]-ATP (3000 Ci/mmol, 10 mCi/mL)   2 μl
- ddH$_2$O   5 μl

2. Incubate at 37°C for 30 min and stop reaction by adding 2 μl 0.5 M EDTA.

3. Add 89 μl TE buffer. Remove an aliquot for percent incorporation (Steps 4 through 9) or proceed with removal of unincorporated nucleotide (Steps 10 through 15).

Determination of percent incorporation

4. Spot 1 μl of the labeled primer onto each of four Whatman DE81 (or equivalent) 2.3 cm circular filters.

5. Dry the filters briefly under a heat lamp. Place two filters aside for direct determination of total cpm in the sample.

6. To remove unincorporated nucleotides, wash the other two filters in 50 mL 0.5 M Na$_2$HPO$_4$, pH 6.8, twice for 5 min each.

7. Dry the washed filters under a heat lamp.

8. Place the filters into individual vials, add cocktail, and determine counts per minute in a scintillation counter.

9. Calculate the average cpm for the total and incorporated filters and calculate percent incorporation. Typically, 50% of the radioactivity is incorporated in the 5′ end labeling reaction.

Removal of unincorporated nucleotide

10. Add 25 μl 5 M ammonium acetate and mix.

11. To this sample, add 200 μl 100% ethanol. Mix and place at –20°C for 30 min.

12. Centrifuge at 12,000 × g for 10 minutes. Carefully remove supernatant.

13. Resuspend pellet in 100 μl 1M ammonium acetate and mix.

14. Ethanol precipitate as described in Steps 10 through 12 above.

15. Dry the pellet under vacuum and resuspend the DNA in 50 μl ddH$_2$O. Count 1 μl of the oligonucleotide and measure the absorbance at 260 nm to determine the concentration of primer. Dilute the primer to 10 pmol/μl in ddH$_2$0

2. PCR Amplification

In these PCR reactions, a constant amount of internal standard is added to each tube. The amount of IS added is not critical as long as it may be easily detected and does not reach a plateau during the amplification. Previous experiments may be required to determine an approximate range to be used.

1. Dilute the internal standard to appropriate concentration for the samples being examined.

Analysis of Gene Expression

Note: *Internal standards are small molecules that can easily become airborne and contaminate future experiments. Whenever possible, utilize aerosol barrier tips and work in a well-ventilated area. Be very careful when handling rcRNA and always keep on ice to prevent degradation. The diluted rcRNA may be stored at $-20°C$, while the stock solutions should be maintained at $-80°C$, in aliquots if necessary, to prevent frequent freeze–thaw cycles.*

Use the following worksheet to prepare the cDNA mix. Multiply the 1X volumes by the number of samples to be examined.

Component	Final Concentration	1X	nX
ddH$_2$O	—	10.5	
MgCl$_2$ (25 mM)	5 mM	4	
10X PCR Buffer	1X	2	
dATP (100 mM)	1 mM	0.2	
dCTP (100 mM)	1 mM	0.2	
dGTP (100 mM)	1 mM	0.2	
dTTP (100 mM)	1 mM	0.2	
Oligo(dT)$_{15}$ (0.5 mg/ml)*	6 μg/ml	0.25	
rRNasin (30 U/μl)	7.5 U	0.25	
Internal standard**	?	2	

* Random hexamers may be substituted for Oligo(dT)$_{15}$.
** This must be determined from previous studies. Use an IS concentration that can be detected at low cycles but does not plateau at high cycles.

2. On ice, add 2 μl of RNA samples (50 ng/μl) to individual PCR tubes.
3. Add the equivalent of 0.3 μl per tube of MMLV reverse transcriptase to the cDNA mix. That is, if there are 25 samples to be examined, add 7.5 μl reverse transcriptase to Mix B.
4. On ice, add 18 μl cDNA mix to the PCR tubes containing the samples, vortex.
5. Place in the thermocycler and run the following program:

42°C for 15 min
95°C for 5 min
Store at 4°C

80   PCR Protocols in Molecular Toxicology

6. While the cDNA synthesis is proceeding, assemble the PCR mixture as follows, at room temperature. The PCR mix is the same for the standard curve and the samples.

Component	Final Concentration (in PCR reaction)*	1X	nX
ddH_2O**	—		22
$MgCl_2$ (25 mM)**	4 mM	4	
10X PCR Buffer	1X	3	
Forward primer (10 pmol/μl)***	6 pmol	0.6	
Reverse primer (10 pmol/μl)***	6 pmol	0.6	

*   The cDNA reaction contains nucleotides, additional $MgCl_2$, and 10X buffer. The final concentration of nucleotides is 400 μM.

** Must be optimized for each primer pair. The example given (4 mM $MgCl_2$) is adequate for most PCR reactions.

*** Either or both of the primers are ^{32}P-labeled as discussed above.

7. When the cDNA reaction is complete, choose one of two methods for assembly of the PCR reaction: hot start (Steps 8 through 11) or cold start (Steps 13 through 16).

Note: Two different methods can be used in an attempt to decrease mispriming and primer artifacts and to assure that all the tubes will start amplification simultaneously. In a hot start all the reagents (cDNA reactions, PCR master mix) are brought to 85°C prior to the addition of Taq. This will prevent the primers from binding to each other and will also dissociate the primers from the template. The easiest way to perform a hot start is to use a heat block that will hold the standard PCR tube. In a cold start the cDNA and the PCR mix are placed on ice. This method is technically easier, and there is less chance of contamination, but the efficiency of amplification is much less than when using a hot start.

Hot Start

8. Immediately prior to completion of the cDNA reaction, place the mix prepared in Step 6 in an 85°C heat block (3 to 5 min).

9. At the completion of the cDNA reaction, remove the tubes from the thermocycler and place them in an 85°C heat block. (The thermocycler may also be used as a surrogate heat block). Add the equivalent of 0.25 μl per tube of Taq DNA polymerase (5 U/μl) to the preheated mix. Vortex and return to the heat block.

Analysis of Gene Expression   **81**

10. Add 30 µl PCR mix directly to the tube containing the cDNA reaction, in the heat block. Work quickly to avoid volatilization.

11. Place the reactions in the thermocycler only when it has reached at least 85°C. A sample PCR reaction is given below. The temperature, times, and cycles must be optimized for each primer pair.

Denature	94°C 4 min
	Cycle (30X)
Denature	94°C 20 sec
Anneal	59°C 30 sec
Elongate	72°C 30 sec
Elongate	72°C 5 min
Store	4°C

12. After cycles 20, 22, 24, 26, 28, and 30, pause the PCR machine. Remove one tube per sample and place on ice.

Note: *Many PCR machines have the capability to automatically pause at the end of the designated cycles. If not, the thermocycler may be manually paused, but wait until the machine has completed the elongation step.*

Cold Start

13. Prepare the PCR mix as suggested in Step 6. Place on ice.

14. At the completion of the cDNA reaction, remove the tubes from the thermocycler and place them on ice. Add the equivalent of 0.25 µl per tube of *Taq* DNA polymerase (5 U/µl) to the cold mix. Vortex and place back on ice.

15. Add 30 µl PCR mix directly to the tube containing the cDNA reaction, on ice.

16. Place the reactions in the thermocycler and run the optimized PCR program.

17. After cycles 20, 22, 24, 26, 28, and 30, pause the PCR machine. Remove one tube per sample and place on ice.

3.   Detection and Quantitation

1. Add loading dye directly to each sample and resolve PCR products as discussed in Chapter 6. Use the thinnest agarose gel possible.

2. Soak the gel in 0.4 N NaOH for 30 minutes and subsequently place in one gel volume of 0.4 N NaOH.

3. Prewet a nylon filter in ddH$_2$O and place on top of gel. Two pieces of filter paper are placed on top of the nylon filter followed by a stack of paper towels. A light weight (1 to 2 kg) is placed on top of the stack and left overnight.

4. Carefully remove the paper towels and filter paper and wrap the nylon filter in plastic wrap.

5. Quantitate the bands by autoradiography or densitometry.

6. Plot $\log(Y_T/Y_S)$ versus n, and solve for the y intercept, $\log(A_T/A_S)$. Multiply A_T/A_S by the amount of IS spiked into the reactions to solve for A_T, the amount of starting target mRNA.

V.   Semiquantitative RT–PCR

A.   Basic Considerations

Semiquantitative RT–PCR, also called coamplification or external standard RT–PCR, requires the amplification of a so-called housekeeping gene concurrently with the target gene.[18,19] The expression of the target gene is expressed relative to that of the reference gene. The reference gene, i.e., the housekeeping gene, is sometimes referred to as an external standard, as it does not control for the amplification efficiency of the target gene itself. Rather, the external standard controls for tube-to-tube differences in the amount of RNA being examined. The housekeeping gene is usually a structural gene such as β-actin and tubulin, or it may be a constitutively expressed enzyme such as glyceraldehyde phosphate dehydrogenase (GAPDH) or hypopurine ribose transferase (HPRT). The key feature of the reference gene is that it cannot be affected by your particular treatment. Therefore, care should be taken in selecting an external standard appropriate for the treatment and tissue of interest.

The semiquantitative, external standard approach has several advantages over the internal standard methods discussed above. For example, a recombinant RNA molecule does not need to be synthesized, quantitation is quite simple, and many samples can be examined simultaneously. However, the external standard procedure is not as sensitive (i.e., it requires a large difference), expresses target gene levels in relative, nonquantitative terms, and is not fully adaptable to every gene of interest.

The protocols listed below are appropriate for a reference gene and a target gene that are being expressed at roughly equivalent levels. If several genes of different expression levels are important (low, medium, and high copy number genes), it is necessary to change reference genes. That is, for a low copy number target gene, use an external standard which is present at low levels in your samples.

Analysis of Gene Expression

B.   Semiquantitative, External Standard RT–PCR

Protocol

1. Prepare the following for the first-strand cDNA synthesis and place on ice. (The final reaction volume will be 20 µl).

Component	Final Concentration	1X	nX
ddH$_2$O	—	10.5	
MgCl$_2$ (25 mM)	5 mM	4	
10X PCR Buffer	1X	2	
dATP (100 mM)	1 mM	0.2	
dCTP (100 mM)	1 mM	0.2	
dGTP (100 mM)	1 mM	0.2	
dTTP (100 mM)	1 mM	0.2	
Oligo(dT)$_{15}$ (0.5 mg/ml)*	6 µg/ml	0.25	
rRNasin (30 U/µl)	7.5 U	0.25	

* Random hexamers may be substituted for Oligo(dT)$_{15}$

2. On ice, add 2 µl of RNA sample (diluted to 0.05 µg/µl) to each tube (100 ng/tube total).

3. Add 2.5 µl (500 U) MMLV reverse transcriptase to the cDNA mixture. Vortex.

Note: *MMLV is the most common type of reverse transcriptase used in cDNA synthesis. AMV reverse transcriptase may be substituted, but use 5 units/tube.*

4. Add 18 µl cDNA mix to the PCR tubes containing the RNA. Cap tubes and vortex briefly to mix.

5. Place in the thermocycler and run the following program:

42°C for 15 min
95°C for 5 min
Store at 4°C

6. While the cDNA synthesis is proceeding, assemble the PCR mixture as follows, at room temperature.

Component	Final Concentration (in PCR reaction)*	1X	nX
ddH$_2$O**	—	22	
MgCl$_2$ (25 m*M*)**	4 m*M*	4	
10X PCR Buffer	1X	3	
Target fp (10 pmol/μl)***	10 pmol	1	
Target rp (10 pmol/μl)	10 pmol	1	
Reference fp (10 pmol/μl)	1 pmol	0.1	
Reference rp (10 pmol/μl)	1 pmol	0.1	

* The cDNA reaction contains nucleotides, additional MgCl$_2$, and 10X buffer. The final concentration of nucleotides in 400 μ*M*.

** Must be optimized for each primer pair. The example given (4 m*M* MgCl$_2$) is adequate for most PCR reactions.

*** The concentration of the target and reference primers must be determined empirically. Both PCR products must be easily detected, the ratio of band intensity should remain constant when a dilution series of RNA is examined, and known stimuli of target gene expression should be examined to determine if the PCR conditions are optimal.

7. When cDNA reaction is complete choose one of two methods for assembly of the PCR reaction: hot start (Steps 8 through 11) or cold start (Steps 12 through 14).

Note: *Two different methods can be used in an attempt to decrease mispriming and primer artifacts and to ensure that all the tubes will start amplification simultaneously. In a hot start all the reagents (cDNA reactions, PCR master mix) are brought to 85°C prior to the addition of* Taq. *This will prevent the primers from binding to each other and will also dissociate the primers from the template. The easiest way to perform a hot start is to use a heat block that will hold the standard PCR tube. In a cold start the cDNA and the PCR mix are placed on ice. This method is technically easier, and there is less chance of contamination, but the efficiency of amplification is much less than when using a hot start.*

Hot Start

8. Immediately prior to completion of the cDNA reaction, place the mix prepared in Step 6 in an 85°C heat block (3 to 5 minutes).

Analysis of Gene Expression

9. At the completion of the cDNA reaction, remove the tubes from the thermocycler and place them in an 85°C heat block. (The thermocycler may also be used as a surrogate heat block). Add 2.5 µl *Taq* DNA polymerase (5 U/µl) to the preheated mix. Vortex and return to the heat block.

10. Add 30 µl PCR mix directly to the tube containing the cDNA reaction in the heat block. Work quickly to avoid evaporation.

11. Place the reactions in the thermocycler only when it has reached at least 85°C. A sample PCR reaction is given below. The temperature, times, and cycles must be optimized for each primer pair. In the case of two divergent optimal temperatures with the target and external standard, choose an annealing temperature that works for the target gene, and adjust the amount of primers until both bands are evident.

Denature	94°C 4 min
	<u>Cycle (30X)</u>
Denature	94°C 20 sec
Anneal	55°C 30 sec
Elongate	72°C 30 sec
Elongate	72°C 5 min
Store	4°C

Cold Start

12. Prepare the PCR mix as suggested in Step 6. Place on ice.

13. At the completion of the cDNA reaction, remove the tubes from the thermocycler and place them on ice. Add 2.5 µl *Taq* DNA polymerase (5 U/µl) to the cold mix. Vortex and place back on ice.

14. Add 30 µl PCR mix directly to the tube containing the cDNA reaction on ice.

15. Place the reactions in the thermocycler and run the optimized PCR program.

C. Quantitation

1. After the PCR amplification, proceed with the agarose gel and photography as discussed previously.

2. For each PCR reaction, express the density of the target gene relative to that of the reference, external standard.

VI. Reverse Transcription PCR *In Situ* Hybridization

The ability to assess whether a gene is induced by a particular treatment usually entails examining mRNA derived from a mixture of cells. Depending on the heterogeneity of cells within a tissue, an important toxicological event may be overlooked. That is, responsive cells may be vastly outnumbered by non-responsive cells and an effect of a treatment on a particular gene may be diluted. *In situ* RT–PCR gives the researcher the ability to examine gene expression on a cell-by-cell basis. A basic protocol for performing *in situ* RT–PCR with a relatively simple detection method is given below. For more details on slide preparation and other detection systems compatible with PCR-based assays, the reader is directed to reference 20.

A. Slide Preparation

1. Cut 4-micron sections of paraffin-embedded tissues onto Probe-On slides (Fisher Biotech) or equivalent.

2. Deparaffinize in xylenes 2 × 5 min, then perform the following:
   - 100% ethanol 2 × 3 min
   - 95% ethanol 2 × 3 min
   - 70% ethanol 2 × 3 min
   - Place slides in TBS buffer

3. Sections are treated with trypsin for 15 min. Prepare trypsin stock and diluted trypsin solution as shown below.
   - Make a 0.5% stock (from Gibco 2.5% Trypsin) in sterile water and store at 4°C until used.
   - Dilute 10 ml of stock into 50 ml of sterile water and add 50 mg of $CaCl_2$, 250 µl of 1 M Tris (pH 7.5), and 50 µl 1 M NaOH (final pH is 7.8)
   - Preheat for 5 min at 37°C. Place slides in trypsin solution for 15 min at 37°C

4. Wash for 1 min in sterile water then place slides in TBS solution (0.05 M Tris-Cl, 0.15 M NaCl) at room temperature for 5 min.

5. Dip slides in 95% ethanol, then 100%, and allow to air dry.

B. cDNA Synthesis

1. Cover the PCR block with aluminum foil to allow for more even distribution of heat.

2. Prepare master mix, including reverse transcriptase (all at room temperature) and pipet 20 µl onto each section. A small dab of grease is applied to the slide although not too close to the section. This will anchor the cover slip. Put mineral oil around the edges of the slip to seal.

Analysis of Gene Expression

Notes: *Use cover slips that will not go all the way to the edge of the slide (e.g., 22 ~ 30 mm). This is to ensure that mineral oil goes around all edges of the slip and gives a good seal. Some mineral oil will go under the cover slip, but this has not been noted to interfere with the reaction.*

cDNA Synthesis Master Mix

Component	Per Slide	Final Concentration
MgCl$_2$ (25 mM)	8 µl	10 mM
10X PCR Buffer	2 µl	1X
dATP (100 mM)	0.2 µl	1 mM
dCTP (100 mM)	0.2 µl	1 mM
dGTP (100 mM)	0.2 µl	1 mM
dTTP (100 mM)	0.2 µl	1 mM
Digoxigenin 11-dUTP	0.5 µl	
Oligo(dT)$_{15}$	0.25 µl	6 µg/ml
rRNasin	1.0 µl	30 U
ddH$_2$O	5.6 µl	
MMLV RT	0.5 µl	100 U

3. Incubate in PCR machine at 42°C for 30 min and allow slides to return to room temperature.

4. Remove cover slip and oil by placing in xylenes. Rinse slides 2 × 3 min in 100% ethanol and allow to air dry.

C. PCR Amplification

1. Warm thermocycler to 85°C using a soak file or hold file. Place one tube of oil per slide in thermocycler or heat block to warm up.

2. Make the PCR mix as suggested below.

Component	Per Slide	Final Concentration
MgCl$_2$ (25 mM)	7.2 µl	9 mM
10X PCR Buffer	2.0 µl	1X
ddH$_2$O	8.3 µl	
Forward primer (10 pmol/µl)	1.0 µl	10 pmol
Reverse primer (10 pmol/µl)	1.0 µl	10 pmol

88   PCR Protocols in Molecular Toxicology

3. Place slides and mix, minus *Taq,* in thermocycler for 1 min.

4. Add 0.5 µl/slide *Taq* DNA polymerase to the mix and quickly pipet 20 µl of mix onto the sections, one at a time (to prevent evaporation). Seal as before.

5. Run the optimal PCR profile as determined from RNA samples obtained from the same tissue.

6. After amplification, remove cover slip and oil in xylenes. Rinse as follows: 100% ethanol (2 × 3 min) then 95, 70, and 50% (2 × 3 min).
   - 100% ethanol 2 × 3 min
   - 95% ethanol 2 × 3 min
   - 70% ethanol 2 × 3 min
   - 50% ethanol 2 × 3 min

Place in TBS buffer. Do not allow slides to dry out.

D.   Signal Detection

1. A Digoxigenin Detection Kit (Boehringer Mannheim, cat# 1210-220) or equivalent may be used.

Steps 1 through 5 are done with gentle agitation:

1. Rinse slides in TBS (0.05 M Tris-Cl, 0.15 M NaCl).
2. Place slides in blocking agent 30 min at room temperature or overnight at 4°C.
3. Wash slides three times 5 to 10 min in TBS.
4. Incubate slides with Antibody (vial 1) at 10 µl per 5 ml TBS for 1 h at room temperature.
5. Wash 2× in TBS and 1 time in TBS-MS, pH 9.5 (0.1 M Tris-Cl, pH 9.5; 0.05 M MgCl$_2$; 0.1 M NaCl) for 5 to 10 min.
6. Staining reaction (mix just prior to use):
   25 µl NBT solution (vial 2)
   19 µl x-phosphate solution (vial 3)
   5 ml TBS-MS
   Develop for a few min up to 1 h
7. Stop reaction by rinsing in distilled water.

2. Counterstain in 1% fast green for 5 sec. Rinse in a large volume of distilled water and drain slides.

3. Add 2 drops of Crystal Mount; spread over section and heat at 60 to 65°C on thermocycler for 20 min. Dip in xylenes, add 1 to 2 drops of Permount, then cover slip.

4. Visualize using standard microscopic techniques.

Analysis of Gene Expression

VII. Analysis of Transcription Rate

A. General Considerations

The analysis of the rate of transcription is an important first step in understanding how a gene is regulated. The accumulation of mRNA can be the result of various events, such as increased transcription, increased stability, decreased breakdown or altered processing. Therefore, increased mRNA levels and increased transcription are not necessarily synonymous. The study of gene transcription is often accomplished by nuclear run-on assays. In this technique, intact nuclei are isolated from control and treated cells. Subsequently, the nuclei are incubated with a radiolabeled nucleic acid to allow the labeling of nascent mRNA. Gene-specific rates of transcription are accomplished by dot- or slot-blotting.

There are obvious limitations in nuclear run-on assays, including the need for large numbers of cells to obtain sufficient nuclei, the use of large amounts of radioactivity, and the relative insensitivity of hybridization detection of transcripts. These problems can be circumvented by utilizing a novel RT–PCR method whereby heterogeneous nuclear RNA is quantitated.[21] Heterogeneous nuclear RNA (hnRNA) are unspliced transcripts, and the following methods take advantage of the fact that this subpopulation of RNA contains intron sequences. The basic procedure is shown in Figure 2.11. In order to quantitate hnRNA, at least one of the primer sequences should be contained within an intron. Also, since hnRNA are relatively large, the distance from the polyadenylation site may be quite far, and reverse transcription may be difficult. Therefore, one can select for a certain population of RNA by using a gene-specific primer for reverse transcription. This reverse transcription primer (RTase primer) may be the same as the reverse PCR primer or may be a nested primer. The latter approach may have increased specificity, but if the nested primer is used at too high a concentration in the RT step, spurious bands may appear upon PCR. Any of the methods described above for constructing an internal standard may be used, although the synthetic standard is depicted.

B. Protocol

Most methods for quantifying hnRNA are identical to that of mRNA, with the exception of primer design. However, two extra controls should be added to the study design.

Additional Control 1. Genomic DNA contamination must be rigorously avoided, because hnDNA and DNA both contain intron sequences, and the PCR products will be identical in size. All RNA should be examined for DNA contamination. This is easiest to determine by performing RT–PCR on

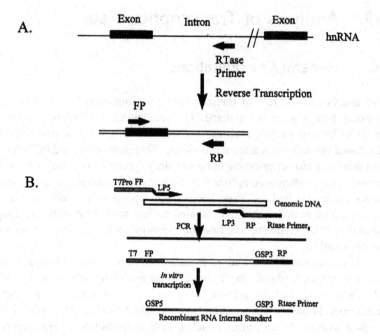

Figure 2.11
Quantitation of heterogeneous nuclear RNA. Panel A. The design of primers for hnRNA examination. The reverse primer should be contained in an intron and can be used in the reverse transcription reaction. The forward primer may be contained within the exon. The reverse transcription primer (RTase primer) may be the same as the reverse PCR primer or may be a nested primer. Panel B. Possible method for synthesizing the internal standard to quantitate hnRNA. The RTase primer and both gene-specific primers are present. This will help to negate tube-to-tube variability in both reverse transcription and PCR.

all samples in parallel, one reaction that receives reverse transcriptase and one that does not. If a PCR product is observed in the absence of reverse transcriptase, DNA contamination is indicated. The RNA may be treated with DNase or may be re-extracted using the methods described in Chapter 6.

Additional Control 2. In order to prove that you are indeed assessing transcription of the target gene, cells or animals treated with a transcription inhibitor such as α-amanitin can be examined. If the induction of hnRNA is not observed in the presence of α-amanitin, transcriptional regulation is implicated.

1. Prepare internal standard using any of the methods described in preceding sections. One of the PCR primers should be within an intron and therefore found in hnRNA but not mRNA.
2. Competitive RT–PCR or cycle-based RT–PCR may be utilized to assess copy number. Substitute RTase primer for Oligo(dT) in the reverse transcriptase reaction.

VIII. Reporter Gene Analysis

A. General Considerations

Reporter gene assays are common laboratory techniques used primarily to examine transcription factor activity. All vectors used in these assays have multiple cloning sites for the introduction of regulatory DNA sequences. These DNA sequences contain promoter or enhancer elements, which in the proper environment will direct transcription of a reporter gene. Common reporter genes are normally not expressed endogenously in mammalian cells and include chloramphenicol acetyltransferase (CAT), β-galactosidase, and luciferase. The expression of each of these reporter genes is assessed by the activity of the enzymes. Luciferase is probably the most common reporter gene used today, and very sensitive and inexpensive assay systems have been developed.

If the enzyme assays for these reporters are so sensitive and simple to perform, why consider PCR at all? The main reason is that measuring the protein product of the reporters is an indirect measure of transcriptional activation. That is, the reporter must be transcriptionally activated, and the mRNA must be translated into protein in an active complex (may require additional cofactors). There have been several studies that have shown that reporter proteins such as luciferase may be regulated through RNA stability or by posttranslational mechanisms. Therefore, the assessment of reporter mRNA levels may be a more direct estimation of transcriptional activity. RT–PCR is easily the most sensitive measure of mRNA production. The measurement of reporter gene mRNA by RT–PCR is very similar to the examination of endogenous mRNA quantitation. The only significant difference is being able to assess the extent of the plasmid DNA that was transfected into the host cells.

Two distinct methods for examination of luciferase mRNA levels are discussed. For a description of transfection procedures, see Chapter 6.

B. Protocol 1

For a review of the procedure, see reference 22.

1. Cotransfect cells with the reporter gene construct containing the DNA sequence of interest (i.e., luciferase reporter) plus a control plasmid (i.e., β-gal). The control plasmid should have a constitutive level of expression and is used to account for differences in transfection efficiency. The ratio of two plasmids may need to be adjusted for optimal transfection efficiency.

2. If response to a particular treatment is to be examined, allow at least 24 h after transfection for the cells to recover. The time of treatment should be adequate for reporter gene mRNA to accumulate.

3. Isolate total RNA directly from the tissue culture plates as discussed in Chapter 6.

92   PCR Protocols in Molecular Toxicology

4. Dilute total RNA to 0.05 µg/µl and perform a standard coamplification or
    external standard RT–PCR (See Section V, this chapter). Prepare the following
    for the first-strand cDNA synthesis and place on ice. (The final reaction volume
    will be 20 µl.)

Component	Final Concentration	1X	nX
ddH$_2$O	—	10.5	
MgCl$_2$ (25 mM)	5 mM	4	
10X PCR Buffer	1X	2	
dATP (100 mM)	1 mM	0.2	
dCTP (100 mM)	1 mM	0.2	
dGTP (100 mM)	1 mM	0.2	
dTTP (100 mM)	1 mM	0.2	
Oligo(dT)$_{15}$ (0.5 mg/ml)*	6 µg/ml	0.25	
rRNasin (30 U/µl)	7.5 U	0.25	

* Random hexamers may be substituted for Oligo(dT)$_{15}$.

5. On ice, add 2 µl of RNA sample (diluted to 0.05 µg/µl) to each tube (100 ng/tube
    total).
6. Add 2.5 µl (500 U) MMLV reverse transcriptase to the cDNA mixture. Vortex.

Note: *MMLV is the most common type of reverse transcriptase used in
          cDNA synthesis. AMV reverse transcriptase may be substituted, but
          use 5 units/tube.*

7. Add 18 µl cDNA mix to the PCR tubes containing the RNA. Cap tubes and
    vortex briefly to mix.
8. Place in the thermocycler and run the following program:

42°C for 15 min
95°C for 5 min
Store at 4°C

9. While the cDNA synthesis is proceeding, assemble the PCR mixture as follows,
    at room temperature.

Component	Final Concentration (in PCR reaction)*	1X	nX
ddH$_2$O**	—	22	

Analysis of Gene Expression

MgCl₂ (25 mM)**	4 mM	4
10X PCR Buffer	1X	3
Reporter fp (10 pmol/µl)***	10 pmol	1
Reporter rp (10 pmol/µl)	10 pmol	1
Control fp (10 pmol/µl)	1 pmol	0.1
Control rp (10 pmol/µl)	1 pmol	0.1

* The cDNA reaction contains nucleotides, additional MgCl₂, and 10X buffer. The final concentration of nucleotides is 400 µM.

** Must be optimized for each primer pair. The example given (4 mM MgCl₂) is adequate for most PCR reactions.

*** The concentration of the target and reference primers must be determined empirically. Both PCR products must be easily detected, the ratio of band intensity should remain constant when a dilution series of RNA is examined, and known stimuli of target gene expression should be examined to determine if the PCR conditions are optimal. The reporter and control primers should be selected from portions of the plasmid that will be transcribed into mRNA. In general, it is best to pick primers that are clearly in the coding sequence of the reporter (i.e., luciferase) and in the control (β-galactosidase).

10. At the completion of the cDNA reaction, remove the tubes from the thermocycler and place them on ice. Add 2.5 µl *Taq* DNA polymerase (5 U/µl) to the cold PCR mix prepared in Step 9. Vortex and place back on ice.

11. Add 30 µl PCR mix directly to the tube containing the cDNA reaction on ice.

12. Place the reactions in the thermocycler and run the optimized PCR program.

13. After the PCR amplification, proceed with the agarose gel and photography as discussed previously.

14. For each PCR reaction, express the density of the target gene product relative to that of the reference, external standard.

C. Protocol 2

In the previous protocol, transfection efficiency was estimated by cotransfecting with control plasmid. This is similar to how reporter assays are performed when enzyme activity is the end point. However, there is some difficulty in determining the ratio of the cotransfected plasmids for optimal activity and amplifying two genes simultaneously requires a fair amount of adjustment.

In the present protocol, primers are designed to detect reporter plasmid DNA as well as the reporter gene mRNA. An outline depicting primer design

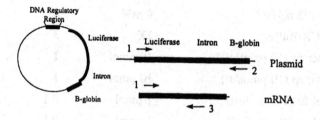

Luciferase primers
(For use with plasmid pGL2 (Promega Corp)
Primer 1: 5' AACATCTTCGACGCGGGCGTG 3'
Primer 2: 5' GCACAATAACCATGCACGTTGCC 3'
Primer 3: 5' GCACGTTGCCCAGGAGCCTG 3'

Figure 2.12
Design of PCR primers for examining luciferase expression.

is shown in Figure 2.12, using luciferase as an example.[23] The reporter gene should contain an intron so when mRNA processing occurs, the plasmid and message PCR products will be distinguishable. Several commercially available reporter vectors have included sequences designed to increase the stability and translation efficiency of the protein. For example, in the case of the luciferase vector pGL2, a small portion of exon 2, a 573 bp intron, and exon 3 of the rabbit β-globin gene have been included. The forward primer 1 and reverse primer 2 are designed to amplify across the intron. In contrast, the reverse primer 3 lies on the boundary of β-globin exon 2 and exon 3. Therefore, this primer will be specific for the messenger RNA and will not amplify from the plasmid. By using two different sets of primers, reporter gene expression and transfection efficiency may be assessed. Internal standards may be designed to quantitate the PCR products derived from primers 1 and 2 as well as from primers 1 and 3. Proceed with the standard quantitative RT-PCR protocols described previously in this chapter (Sections II–IV).

Reagents Needed

Any of the PCR buffers may be used in PCR. Buffer A may be used in both reverse transcriptase and PCR steps.

10X PCR Buffer A

670 mM Tris-HCl, pH 8.8
160 mM $(NH_4)_2SO_4$
8 μM EDTA
3% β-mercaptoethanol
1 mg/ml bovine serum albumin (nuclease free)

Analysis of Gene Expression

10X PCR Buffer B

500 mM KCl
100 mM Tris-HCl, pH 9.0 (at 25°C)
1.0% Triton X-100

10X PCR Buffer C

100 mM Tris-HCl, pH 8.3
500 mM KCl
0.1% BSA

5X MMLV Buffer

250 mM Tris-HCl, pH 8.3
375 mM KCl
15 mM MgCl$_2$

10X Transcription Buffer

800 mM HEPES-KOH, pH 7.5
240 mM MgCl$_2$
20 mM Spermidine
400 mM DTT

10X Ligase Buffer

300 mM Tris-HCl, pH 7.8
100 mM MgCl$_2$
100 mM DTT
10 mM ATP

10X Forward Exchange Buffer

0.5 M Tris-HCl, pH 7.5
0.1 M MgCl$_2$
50 mM DTT
1 mM Spermidine

TE Buffer

10 mM Tris-HCl, pH 8.0
1 mM EDTA

0.5 M EDTA

Chloroform/phenol (1:1)

Mix equal parts TE buffer and phenol and allow phases to separate. Then mix 1 part of the lower phenol phase with one part chloroform. Store in dark at 4°C

PCR Primers

Dilute stock primers to 100 pmol/μl in ddH$_2$O and store at –70°C

For a working stock, dilute to 10 pmol/μl and store at –20°C

10X Ficoll Loading Buffer

30% Ficoll in TE buffer
0.25% Bromophenol blue
0.25% Xylene cyanol (optional)

References

1. **Sewall, C.H., Bell, D.A., Clark, G.C., Tritscher, A.M., Tully, D., Vanden Heuvel, J., and Lucier, G.W.**, Induced gene transcription: Implications for biomarkers, *Clin. Chem.*, 41, 1829, 1995.
2. **Tritscher, A.M., Clark, G.C., Vanden Heuvel, J.P., Sewall, C.H., and Lucier, G.W.**, Tumor promotion by 2,3,7,8-TCDD: Identification of biomarkers and characterization of dose-response relationships, *Organohalogen Compd.*, 13, 167, 1993.
3. **Becker-André, M.**, Absolute levels of mRNA by polymerase chain reaction-aided transcript titration assay, *Meth. Enzymol.*, 218, 420, 1993.
4. **Becker-André, M.**, PCR-aided transcript titration assay: Competitive PCR for evaluation of absolute levels of rare mRNA species, *Meth. Neurosci.*, 26, 129, 1995.
5. **Gilliland, G.S., Perrin, K., and Bunn, H.F.**, Competitive PCR for quantitation of mRNA, in *PCR Protocols: A Guide to Methods and Applications*, Innis et al., Eds., Academic Press, San Diego, 1990, 60.
6. **Mohler, K.M. and Butler, L.D.**, Quantitation of cytokine mRNA levels utilizing the reverse transcriptase-polymerase chain reaction following primary antigen-specific sensitization in vivo-I. Verification of linearity, reproducibility and specificity, *Molec. Immunol.*, 28, 437, 1991.
7. **Nedelman, J., Heagerty, P., and Lawrence, C.**, Quantitative PCR with internal controls, *CABIOS*, 8, 65, 1992.
8. **Sur, S., Gleich, G.J., Bolander, M.E., and Sarkar, G.**, Comparative evaluation of quantitative PCR methods, *Meth. Neurosci.*, 26, 147, 1995.
9. **Volkenandt, M., Dicker, A.P., Banerjee, D., Fanin, R., Schweitzer, Horikoshi, T., Danenberg, K., Danenberg, P., and Bertino, J.R.**, Quantitation of gene copy number and mRNA using the polymerase chain reaction, *Proc. Soc. Exp. Biol. Med.*, 200, 1, 1992.

Analysis of Gene Expression

10. **Vanden Heuvel, J.P., Tyson, F.L., and Bell, D.A.,** Constructions of recombinant RNA templates for use as internal standards in quantitative RT–PCR, *BioTechniques,* 14, 395, 1993.

11. **Ansaldi, M., Lepelletier, M., and Mejean, V.,** Site-specific mutagenesis by using an accurate recombinant polymerase chain reaction method, *Anal. Biochem.,* 234, 110, 1996.

12. **Finney, M., Nisson, P.E., and Rachtchian, A.,** Molecular Cloning of PCR Products, *Current Protocols in Molecular Biology,* 15.7.1, 1995.

13. **Sambrook, J., Fritsch, E.F., and Maniatis, T.,** *Molecular Cloning, A Laboratory Manual,* 2nd ed., Cold Spring Harbor Press, Cold Spring Harbor, NY, 1989.

14. **Sterchele, P.F., Sun, H., Peterson, R.E., and Vanden Heuvel, J.P.,** Regulation of peroxisome proliferator-activated receptor-α mRNA in rat liver, *Arch. Biochem. Biophys.,* 326, 281, 1996.

15. **Zachar, V., Thomas, R.A., and Goustin, A.S.,** Absolute quantification of target DNA: A simple competitive PCR for efficient analysis of multiple samples, *Nucl. Acids Res.,* 21, 2017, 1993.

16. **Vanden Heuvel, J.P., Clark, G.C., Kohn, M.C., Tritscher, A.M., Greenlee, W.F., Lucier, G.W., and Bell, D.A.,** Dioxin-responsive genes: Examination of dose-response relationships using quantitative reverse transcriptase-polymerase chain reaction, *Cancer Res.,* 54, 62, 1994.

17. **Vanden Heuvel, J.P., Clark, G.C., Thompson, C.L., McCoy, Z., Miller, C.R., Lucier, G.W., and Bell, D.A.,** CYP1A1 mRNA levels as a human exposure biomarker: Use of quantitative polymerase chain reaction to measure CYP1A1 expression in human peripheral blood lymphocytes, *Carcinogenesis,* 14, 2003, 1993.

18. **Kaufman, P.B., Wu, W., Kim, D., and Cseke, L.J.,** Analysis of gene expression by semiquantitative PCR, in *Molecular and Cellular Methods in Biology and Medicine,* CRC Press, Boca Raton., FL, 1995, 245.

19. **Scheuermann, R.H. and Bauer, S.R.,** Polymerase chain reaction-based mRNA quantification using an internal standard: Analysis of oncogene expression, *Methods Enzymology,* 218, 446.

20. **O'Leary, J.J., Chetty, R., Graham, A.K., and McGee, J. O'D.,** In situ PCR: Pathologists dream or nightmare?, *J. Pathol.,* 178, 11, 1996.

21. **Elferink, C.J. and Reiners, J.J.,** Quantitative RT–PCR on CYP1A1 heterogenous nuclear RNA: A surrogate for the in vitro transcription run-on assay, *Biotechniques,* 20, 470, 1996.

22. **Kawamoto, S.,** Evidence for an internal regulatory region in a human nonmuscle myosin heavy chain gene, *J. Biol. Chem.,* 269, 15101, 1994.

23. **Kastenbauer, S., Wedel, A., Frankenberger, M., Wirth, T., and Ziegler-Heitbrock, H.W.L.,** Analysis of promoter activity by polymerase chain reaction amplification of reporter gene mRNA, *Anal. Biochem.,* 233, 137, 1996.

Chapter 3

Differential Display PCR

J. Christopher Corton

Contents

I.   General Strategies and Applications...99
II.   Liang and Pardee Method..103
    A.   Preparation of Total or Poly(A) RNA....................................103
    B.   Reverse Transcription...104
    C.   PCR Amplification..106
III.   Sokolov and Prockop Method..107
    A.   Sample Preparation...107
    B.   cDNA Synthesis..108
    C.   PCR Amplification..108
    D.   Gel Electrophoresis...109
IV.   Cloning Differential Display Fragments and Confirmation of
    Altered Expression...109
    A.   Reamplification of cDNA Fragment......................................109
    B.   Cloning Amplified Fragments...110
    C.   Confirmation of Size of Insert by Colony-PCR....................112
    D.   Confirmation of Altered Expression by Dot-Blot Differential
        Hybridization...113
Reagents Needed...115
References..117

I.   General Strategies and Applications

Differential gene expression occurs in the process of carcinogenesis, apoptosis, cellular injury, development, and differentiation. Since all of these complex states are of vital importance to the molecular toxicologist, identifying differentially expressed mRNAs has become a major undertaking in many laboratories. The most common methods employed to compare steady-state mRNA concentrations includes differential or subtractive hybridization (SH), electronic subtraction (ES, also called serial analysis of gene expression or SAGE), and differential display (DD) polymerase chain reaction. Each of these methods has several advantages and disadvantages and all are technically challenging. Recently, the first side-by-side comparison of SH, ES, and DD was performed[1] to determine which method is most reliable. These authors concluded that DD is the method of choice because it can identify low expression mRNAs in a small amount of sample and is able to recognize induced as well as repressed genes in a short period of time.

In this chapter, we will discuss the PCR-based, differential display. The first section describes the original differential display technique of Liang and Pardee[2] used to identify mRNA species of differentially expressed genes. Short DNA sequences (<800 bp) corresponding to these mRNAs can be recovered, cloned, sequenced, and used as Northern blot hybridization or library screening probes. The basic principle illustrated in Figure 3.1 is to reverse transcribe a subpopulation of mRNAs with sets of anchored oligo(dT) primers ($T_{12}MN$ or $T_{12}VN$, where M can be dG, dA, and dC; N is dG, dA, dT, or dC; and V is dG, dA, or dC). The resulting cDNA population is PCR-amplified using the oligo(dT) primer and an arbitrary decamer primer in the presence of radioactive nucleotide. The labeled PCR products are separated on denaturing polyacrylamide gels. By changing primer combinations, most of the RNA species in a cell may be represented. Side-by-side comparison of RNA samples from cells or tissues from two or more treatment groups allows the identification and cloning of differentially expressed genes. Another method, RNA fingerprinting, is similar to differential display but uses one or more arbitrary primers (reviewed by McClellan et al.[3]).

After electrophoresis, bands of interest are cut from the polyacrylamide gel and used as templates in amplification reactions to obtain microgram quantities of the fragment for cloning (Figure 3.2). Once the fragment has been cloned, altered expression can be confirmed by a number of techniques. For small numbers of fragments isolated, each cloned fragment can be used as a probe in slot-blot or conventional Northern blot hybridization. Larger numbers of fragments can be handled in an expeditious manner following a dot-blot differential hybridization procedure,[4] as discussed in the latter portions of this chapter. Briefly, after the amplified fragments are cloned into a T-tailed vector, colonies are picked, transferred to 150-mm plates premarked in a 96-well format, and used directly as a source of template in colony-PCR. Inserts of the correct size are identified by agarose gel electrophoresis. Those colonies that contain the cloned fragments of interest are individually spotted onto a 150-mm master agar plate containing appropriate antibiotics, allowed to grow, and then used as a source of template in another amplification reaction. Equal amounts of the amplified fragments are then dot-blotted onto duplicate filters, which are probed with [^{32}P]-labeled cDNAs from control and treated tissues.

Differential Display PCR

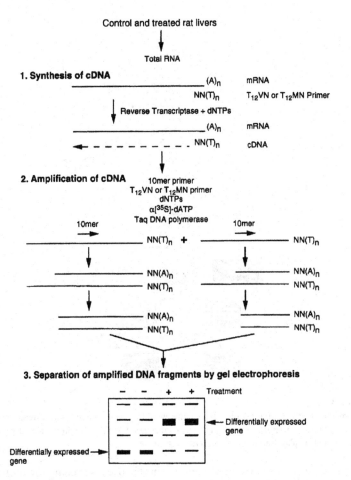

Figure 3.1
Differential display.

Filters are compared for changes in the intensity of the dots after exposure. Once altered expression has been confirmed, the cloned fragments can be sequenced to identify the gene from which they are derived, used to characterize mRNA expression, or used to probe an appropriate cDNA library to isolate the full-length cDNA. Alternatively, the 5′ and 3′ unknown sequences may be isolated by rapid amplification of cDNA ends[5,6] (RACE; also see Chapter 4).

An alternative to the differential display protocol, introduced by Sokolov and Prockop,[7] allows longer fragments of expressed genes to be visualized and isolated. The Sokolov and Prockop method is discussed in the second section. This method is similar to differential display except that the reverse transcription reaction is performed in the presence of a fully degenerate 6mer oligonucleotide, two to three longer primers are used in the subsequent PCR, and the products of the reaction are visualized on agarose gels. The advantages of this technique over that of differential display are that 1) the time it takes

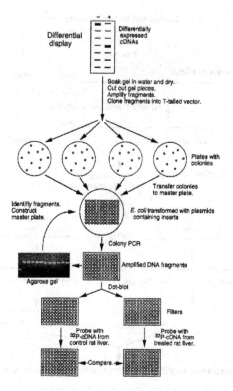

Figure 3.2
Confirmation of altered expression of large numbers of fragments generated by differential display. The procedures for amplification, cloning, and confirmation of altered expression of large numbers of differential display fragments are described in the text.

to go from RNA to cloned fragment is shorter because reamplification of the fragment is not necessary, 2) more sequence information can be generated from the larger differential display fragments (i.e., ≤3000 bp) increasing the chance that the putative open reading frame will be identified in GenBank™ searches, and 3) no radioactivity is used to visualize the fragments. Disadvantages of this technique over differential display include the large number of reactions that need to be performed and the poor resolution of the amplified fragments by agarose gels.

Differential display provides a number of important advantages over alternative differential or subtractive hybridization techniques.[1] 1) Only 20 ng of total RNA are required for each differential display reaction and only a few micrograms to screen over half of the total number of messages. Subtractive hybridization requires 50-fold or more RNA. 2) Differential display bands are visualized in two days and can be cloned in one week. Two months are required to isolate clones from cells by subtractive hybridization. 3) Differential display is less technically demanding. Since the assay can be checked at each step, it is no longer necessary, as with the other methods, to wait until the end of the

Differential Display PCR

procedure to determine whether the procedure worked properly. 4) Unlike subtractive hybridization, which selects for genes that are either more or less abundant, differential display can simultaneously allow for selection of both positive and negative differences unique to a process.

The ability of differential display to visualize rare messages is controversial. An analysis of mRNA species detected by differential display indicates a strong bias toward high copy number mRNAs.[8] On the other hand, a number of groups have claimed that low abundance messages can be easily displayed.[2,9] A large literature database demonstrates the usefulness of this technique in isolating differentially expressed genes, including those that are of interest to toxicologists.

II. Liang and Pardee Method

To get you started, a number of companies sell kits or products for performing differential display (GenHunter Corp., Nashville, TN; Ambion, Austin, TX; Operon Technologies, Alameda, CA; Genomyx, Foster City, CA) or RNA fingerprinting (Clontech, Palo Alto, CA).

A. Preparation of Total or Poly(A) RNA

Note: *Experiments involving RNA require careful technique to prevent RNA degradation.*

Although both total RNA or poly(A) RNA can be used for differential display, total RNA is the template of choice because of its easy isolation and the high background smear problem associated with poly(A) RNA. Total cellular RNA isolation can be carried out using either the standard CsCl gradient[10] or a simplified method developed by Chomczynski and Sacchi.[11] The isolated RNA should be stored in diethyl pyrocarbonate-(DEPC)-treated H_2O or as an ethanol precipitate at $-80°C$.

Differential amounts of contaminating chromosomal DNA in RNA samples can sometimes lead to the identification of false-positive DNA fragments on differential display gels. Although not always necessary, contaminating chromosomal DNA can be removed by digesting the DNA with RNase-free DNase I. The extent of contamination before the DNase reaction can be determined by performing two sets of reverse-transcription and subsequent amplification reactions, one with and one without reverse transcriptase. Fragments that appear in the absence of reverse transcriptase can be attributed to contaminating chromosomal DNA. One reason to avoid the DNase I step, especially if DNA contamination does not affect the display pattern, is that the reaction potentially introduces a point at which the RNA could be unintentionally contaminated and subsequently degraded by RNases.

104   PCR Protocols in Molecular Toxicology

Protocol — Digestion of Contaminating Chromosomal DNA in RNA

1. Digest DNA contaminating total cellular RNA or poly(A) RNA by mixing:

   10 to 100 µg of total RNA

   10 µl 1 U/µl human placental RNase inhibitor

   1 µl 20 U/µl RNase-free DNase I (e.g., Promega, GeneHunter)

   5 µl 0.1 M Tris-Cl, pH 8.3

   5 µl 0.5 M KCl

   5 µL 15 mM MgCl$_2$

   H$_2$O to 50 µl

   Incubate 30 min at 37°C.

2. Add 50 µl phenol/chloroform (3:1), vortex for 30 sec, and leave on ice for 10 min to inactivate DNase I before cDNA synthesis. Separate the phases in a refrigerated microcentrifuge for 5 min at maximum speed.

3. Transfer the upper phase to a microcentrifuge tube and add 5 µl of 3 M sodium acetate and 200 µl of 100% ethanol. Mix and incubate 30 min at –70°C to precipitate RNA.

4. Microcentrifuge (4°C) 15 min at high speed. Carefully pour off supernatant, taking care not to lose the pellet. Wash the pellet once with 500 µl of 70% ethanol (made with DEPC-treated H$_2$O).

5. Dissolve RNA pellet in 20 µl DEPC-treated water and quantitate the RNA concentration by measuring the A_{260} with a UV spectrophotometer. DNA-free RNA should be stored at a concentration >1.1 µg/µl. It should not be diluted to the working concentration until immediately before reverse transcription. Diluted RNA should not be reused for differential display since it is very unstable during storage and after repeated freezing and thawing.

6. Electrophorese 1 to 3 µg of cleaned RNA on a 1% nondenaturing agarose gel or a denaturing 7% formaldehyde agarose gel to check the integrity of the RNA to be used for differential display. For undegraded total RNA, the 28S and 18S ribosomal RNA should be clearly visible by ethidium bromide staining. Store DNA-free RNA at –80°C until used for differential display.

B.   Reverse Transcription

Choice of Primers. Based on theoretical considerations, 12 possible anchored oligo(dT) primers (T_{12}VN where V may be dG, dA, or dC, and N may be any one of the four deoxynucleotides) used in all combinations with at least 20 different arbitrary 10mers are necessary to display 10,000 of the approximately 15,000 mRNA species in a mammalian cell.[2,12] Because the

Differential Display PCR

105

penultimate base V can exhibit considerable degeneracy in the reverse transcriptase reaction,[13] four $T_{12}MN$ primers (where M is degenerate and consists of dG, dA, and dC) can be used to replace the $T_{12}VN$ primers[14] decreasing considerably the number of reactions theoretically necessary to screen the mRNA species.

Any arbitrary decamer or longer can be used in the differential display reaction as long as palindromic sequences are not present and the G+C content is 50 to 70%. Because the arbitrary decamer has been shown to contain up to four bp mismatches with the original DNA templates clustered at the 5' end of the primers,[13] the arbitrary 10mer can be designed such that the 3' ends are maximally randomized. Sets of primers that have been designed with these conditions in mind can be found in Bauer et al.[12] and are commercially available (GenHunter Corp., Nashville, TN; Operon Technologies, Alameda, CA; Genosys Biotechnology, The Woodlands, TX).

Note: *Because of the inherent variability in the differential display procedure, at least two samples from each group should be compared. Only those fragments that are clearly different should be characterized further.*

Protocol — Reverse Transcription

1. Label one 0.5 mL microcentrifuge tube for each oligo(dT) primer.

2. Freshly dilute total RNA or DNA-free total RNA to 0.1 µg/µl in DEPC-treated water and place on ice. Immediately freeze the remaining undiluted RNA sample to avoid degradation.

3. Set up reverse transcription of total RNA with each of the different oligo(dT) primers as follows:

   H_2O to give 19 µl total volume

   4 µl 5 × MMLV reverse transcriptase buffer (1 × final)

   2 µl 0.1 M DTT (10 mM final)

   1.6 µl 250 µM 4dNTP mix (20 µM final)

   2 µl of 0.1 µg/µl total RNA

   2 µl of one 10 µM anchored oligo(dT) primer (1 µM final).

4. Incubate the tubes 5 min at 65°C to denature the mRNA secondary structure and 10 min at 37°C in a thermocycler to allow primer annealing.

5. Add 1 µl of 200 U/µl MMLV reverse transcriptase to each tube, mix well, and incubate 50 min at 37°C.

6. Incubate 5 min at 95°C to inactivate the reverse transcriptase. Microcentrifuge briefly at high speed to collect condensation. Place the tube on ice for immediate PCR amplification or store at –20°C for later use (stable at least 6 months).

C. PCR Amplification

Protocol — PCR Amplification

1. Prepare a 20-µl reaction mix for each primer set as follows:

   9.7 µl H₂O

   2 µl 10 × amplification buffer (1 × final)

   1.6 µl 25 μM 4dNTP mix (2 μM final)

   0.5 µl 10 µCi/µl [α-^{35}S]dATP (1200 Ci/mmole)

   2 µl 2 μM arbitrary decamer (0.2 μM final)

   2 µl 10 μM anchored oligo(dT) primer (1 μM final)

   2 µl cDNA (from reverse transcription protocol)

   0.2 µl 5 U/µl *Taq* DNA polymerase (1 unit).

   Because accurately pipetting 0.2 µl of *Taq* DNA polymerase is difficult, prepare enough stock PCR reaction mix without the arbitrary decamer for the number of reactions to be run plus one, mix well, and aliquot 18 µl to each tube. Add the arbitrary decamer to the appropriate tubes.

2. Tap the tube to mix, spin the contents down briefly in the microfuge, and overlay the sample with 25 µl mineral oil. (When using a Perkin-Elmer 9600 thermocycler or equivalent, mineral oil is not necessary.)

3. Carry out PCR in a thermal cycler using the following amplification cycles:

40 cycles:	30 sec	94°C (denaturation)
	2 min	40°C (annealing)
	30 sec	72°C (extension)
1 cycle:	5 min	72°C (extension)
Final step:	Soak	4°C (hold)

   The 2-min incubation at 40°C allows sufficient time for the short primers to anneal and start extension. The short extension period at 72°C allows for the amplification of only short (<800-bp) DNA products that can be resolved on a denaturing polyacrylamide gel. PCR products may be stored at 4°C or –20°C until used.

4. Mix 3.5 µl PCR product with 2 µl formamide loading buffer and incubate 2 min at 80°C. Load sample onto a 5% denaturing sequencing-type polyacrylamide gel. Run the gel ~3 h at 60 W until the xylene cyanol dye runs to within 1 cm of the bottom. DNA fragments smaller than 130 bp (the mobility of xylene cyanol on a 5% denaturing gel) are more difficult to use as hybridization probes in subsequent analysis and are usually ignored.

5. In a large tray, immerse the gel sitting on one glass plate in ~ 2 cm of distilled H₂O for 15 to 20 min to remove urea. Be careful not to allow gel to float off the glass plate. Lift glass plate out of the water, pour off excess water and transfer gel onto a piece of Whatman 3MM paper. Cover the gel with a sheet of Saran® Wrap and dry under vacuum for 20 to 60 min at 80°C. Remove the Saran Wrap

Differential Display PCR 107

and orient the dried gel with radioactive ink or with autoradiography markers (e.g., Glogos™II, Stratagene; Identi-kit, Diversified Biotech, Newton Center, MA). Expose X-ray film at room temperature for 18 to 48 h. The dried gel should always be handled with gloves to prevent DNA contamination. Store the dried gel between two sheets of clean Whatman 3MM filter paper.

Deviations from protocol. The $\alpha[^{35}S]$-dATP can be substituted with either 0.25 μL $\alpha[^{32}P]$-dATP (200 Ci/mmole) or 1 μL $\alpha[^{33}P]$-dATP (2000 Ci/mmole). Radioactivity has been successfully omitted by a number of groups. Application of the method to an automated DNA sequencer enabled nonradioactive quantitation of differential display fragments.[12] FITC-conjugated primers have been used in the PCR to enable detection of band patterns by a fluorescence image analyzer.[15] Digoxigenin (DIG)-labeled oligonucleotides have been used in the differential display to allow detection of the fragments transferred to nylon membranes by an anti-DIG-alkaline phosphatase antibody–enzyme conjugate.[16] The DNA bands have also been visualized by silver staining.[17]

A number of groups have changed the RT or PCR conditions or both to enable more reliable amplification of longer or increased numbers of products. Guimarães et al.[9] suggested that increasing the 10mer primer concentration to 30 μM and performing the annealing at 32°C for 15 sec increases the number of differential display bands. Linskens et al.[18] found increased numbers of fragments by replacing the 10mer primers with 22 bp primers and performing the amplification for four cycles at a low annealing temperature (41°C) followed by 18 cycles at an annealing temperature of 60°C. The use of an RNase H-deficient reverse transcriptase enabled a better presentation of differentially expressed genes.[19] The differential display and RNA fingerprinting techniques have been combined in a protocol requiring only a single cDNA synthesis for each RNA sample with longer primers, and higher stringency PCR to display bands up to 2 kb.[20] Several groups have replaced the random 10mers with degenerate primers designed to amplify members of the nuclear receptor[21] and Cys_2/His_2 zinc finger[22] families. Differential display has been coupled to subtractive techniques to increase the frequency of isolation of differentially expressed genes.[23]

III.   Sokolov and Prockop Method

These procedures are adapted from the original description of the technique.[7]

A.   Sample Preparation

1. Extract total RNA from tissues/cells of interest using TriReagent (MRC Corp, Cincinnati, OH) according to the manufacturers instructions.[11] Also, see Chapter 6 for alternative RNA extraction methods.

2. Utilizing the total RNA from above, obtain mRNA using PolyATract mRNA Isolation System (Promega Corp., Madison, WI) according to the manufacturer's instructions. Also, see Chapter 6 for alternative polyA extraction methods.

108 PCR Protocols in Molecular Toxicology

3. Dilute mRNA to 100 ng/µl in DEPC-treated water.

B.   cDNA Synthesis

1. Set up the following cDNA reaction. Make a pooled mix for multiple samples.

	1X (µl)	*Final Concentration*
MgCl$_2$ (25 mM)	4	2.5 mM
5X first-strand buffer	8	1X
Random hexamers (50 µM)	1	1.25 µM
RNasin (50 U/µl)	0.5	0.625 U/µL
dNTPs (100 mM)	0.2 each	0.5 mM
Superscript RT (200 U/µl)	1	5 U/µL
mRNA (100 ng/µl)	3	7.5 ng/µL
ddH$_2$O	Up to 40	

2. Using a thermocycler, run the following program:

20°C for 15 min
42°C for 50 min
99°C for 5 min
4°C for 10 min

3. Add 4U RNase H to each tube.

4. Incubate at 37°C for 30 min followed by 65°C for 5 min.

C.   PCR Amplification

1. The total volume of the PCR reaction is 50 µl. The amount of primer and cDNA used may be adjusted. (We have found 20 pmol primer and 4 µl cDNA mix to work well.) Set up the following reaction. Use a hot start if possible.

	1X (µl)	*Final Concentration*
MgCl$_2$ (25 mM)	3	1.5 mM
10X PCR buffer	5	1X

Differential Display PCR

dNTPs (100 mM)	0.1 µl each	0.2 mM
10 pmol/µl "primer X"*	2	0.4 pmol/µL
10 pmol/µl "primer Y"*	2	0.4 pmol/µL
Taq polymerase	1	0.1 U/µL
cDNA reaction	2 to 4	Approx. 0.8 ng/µL
ddH$_2$O	up to 50	

* 10mer of 60% GC content that contain no stop codon. Genosys Biotechnology (The Woodlands, TX) sells kits of 10mers for use in these types of assays.

2. Run the following PCR program:

Hot start at 85°C, then:

95°C	3 min
45 cycles of:	
94.5°C	30 sec
34°C	1 min
72°C	1 min

Followed by:

72°C for 5 min

D. Gel Electrophoresis

Run a 1.5% Metaphor (FMC Corp.) gel with 15 µl sample/lane at 100 V for 2 h.

Differentially expressed bands can be easily excised from the gel and purified as discussed in Chapter 6. Reamplification of the PCR products is not necessary. Proceed with cloning and verification as discussed below.

IV. Cloning Differential Display Fragments and Confirmation of Altered Expression

A. Reamplification of cDNA Fragment

Reamplification is necessary for the Liang and Pardee method. For Sokolov and Prockop, continue with Section B.

110 PCR Protocols in Molecular Toxicology

Protocol — Reamplification of cDNA Fragment

1. Develop the film and photograph or scan the relevant parts of the film before isolation of DNA fragments. Mark DNA bands of interest (those differentially displayed in different lanes) by drawing rectangles around the fragments to be isolated on the film with a heavy black pen.

2. On a light box, secure the dried gel to a clean glass plate. Align the film over the gel and cut out gel slices by cutting through the marked regions on X-ray film. Place a 1 to 2 mm × 1 to 2 mm piece of the gel into a PCR tube and the rest of the isolated fragment into another tube for indefinite storage. Expose film to the cut gel to confirm that the correct band was isolated.

3. To the PCR tube containing the dried gel fragment, add 20 µL of the original PCR mix containing the same oligo(dT) and 10mer primers used to amplify the fragment, except add 1.6 µL of 250 μM 4dNTP mix (20 μM final) instead of 1.6 µL of 25 μM 4dNTP mix and omit the isotope. Be careful to ensure that the gel piece is not protruding through the mineral oil or evaporation will occur. Amplify the fragments using the same PCR conditions as before.

4. Electrophorese 3 µL of each PCR sample on a 1.5% agarose gel prestained with ethidium bromide to check the molecular weight of the fragment.

Note: *If the DNA fragment is not visible after the first reamplification, another aliquot of Taq DNA polymerase can be added and the reaction repeated. The amplified fragments must be kept cold to decrease the chance of loss of the A overhangs by contaminating nucleases, which will seriously decrease cloning efficiency.*

Deviations from protocol. In the original descriptions of DNA isolation from the dried gel, the DNA was eluted in H_2O by boiling, followed by precipitation in the presence of glycogen.[2,13] The pellet was resuspended in 10 µL H_2O, and 4 µL was used in the amplification.

B. Cloning Amplified Fragments

The following protocol was adapted from that provided with the popular TA Cloning® kit (Invitrogen, San Diego, CA) to reduce the amount of plasmid vector (pCRII) and cells required for each ligation and transformation.[4] The plasmid in this kit can be replaced with any T-tailed vector. A protocol for making T-tailed vectors is found in Chapter 4.

Protocol — Cloning Amplified Fragments

1. Set up a series of ligations with different amounts of a test fragment of known concentration and 12.5 ng of the vector pCRII to determine the optimal ratio of fragment to vector. Each ligation reaction should contain:

Differential Display PCR

H$_2$O to 5 μL

1 μL 5 × ligation buffer

1 μL pCRII (diluted to 12.5 ng/μL with H$_2$O)

0 to 2.5 μL of fragment (~10 to 50 ng/μL) at 0.5 μL intervals

0.3 μL of T4 DNA ligase

2. Incubate the reaction at 14 to 15°C for at least 4 h (overnight will increase the number of transformants).

3. Transform 20 μL of competent cells (supplied by TA Cloning kit; transformation efficiency, 1 × 10^8 transformants/μg of supercoiled plasmid) with 2 μL of the ligation. Mix by tapping gently. Cells are prepared by thawing on ice a 50-μL vial of the competent cells followed by the addition of 2 μL of 0.5 μM β-mercaptoethanol, which is stirred into the cells with a pipette tip. Store the remaining ligation mixture(s) at –20°C. Highly competent cells can be made by following the procedures outlined in Ausubel et al.[10]

4. Incubate the transformation mixtures on ice for 30 min.

5. Heat-shock the transformation mixtures at 42°C for exactly 30 sec. Do not mix.

6. Immediately place the tubes on ice for 2 min.

7. Add 180 μL of prewarmed (37°C) SOC medium to each tube. Use good sterile technique to prevent contamination.

8. Place the tubes in a microcentrifuge rack and shake the tubes at 37°C for at least 40 min at 225 rpm in a rotary shaking incubator.

9. While the tubes are shaking, prepare the LB agar plates containing either kanamycin (50 μg/mL) or ampicillin (50 μg/mL) by spreading 25 μL of X-Gal (40 mg/mL stock in dimethylformamide) on top of the agar with a glass spreader. The plates should not be dry to ensure even distribution of the X-Gal. Let the X-Gal diffuse into the agar for at least 30 min.

10. Briefly pellet the cells in a microcentrifuge (at highest setting) for 10 to 15 sec. Pour off most of the supernatant, leaving ~100 to 200 μL of SOC medium over the pellet.

11. Resuspend the pellet by pipetting the SOC medium up and down, breaking up the bacterial pellet.

12. Spread the entire transformation onto a marked LB agar plate containing antibiotic and X-Gal.

13. Invert the plates and place them in a 37°C incubator overnight. In a few cases, a longer incubation may be required to allow the blue color to develop.

14. Determine the optimal ratio of fragment to vector that results in the highest percentage of white colonies. When cloning fragments smaller than ~500 bp, light blue rather than white colonies may appear. In this case, the open reading frame of the *lacZ* gene is still intact. These colonies should be treated as if they were white since they may contain inserts. Check colonies by colony-PCR (described below) for inserts of the correct size. At the optimal ratio of fragment to vector, ~100 to 300 colonies should be observed with 10 to 90% containing plasmids with inserts.

112 PCR Protocols in Molecular Toxicology

15. Repeat the ligation and transformation for the other isolated fragments using the optimal concentration of the test fragment as a guide. To determine the amount of each fragment to add to the ligation reaction, compare on the same agarose gel the amount of test fragment for optimal cloning and equal volumes of the remaining fragments to be cloned.

C. Confirmation of Size of Insert by Colony-PCR

This protocol is a modification of the original colony-PCR technique.[24]

Protocol — Colony-PCR

1. Immediately before amplification, set up PCR tubes (MicroAmp, Perkin Elmer) containing 15 μL of amplification mix.

2. Touch each colony to be analyzed with a sterile pipet tip and spot a 150-mm plate containing YT plus antibiotic premarked in a 96-well format. Place the pipet tip into the corresponding PCR tube containing the amplification mix. When all the tubes are filled, remove the tips before amplification, being careful not to contaminate the adjacent tubes.

3. Perform the amplification in a Perkin Elmer 9600 thermocycler or other thermocycler with a 96-well format as follows:

1 cycle:	5 min	94°C (cell lysis)
25 cycles:	30 sec	94°C (denaturation)
	30 sec	55°C (annealing)
	30 sec	72°C (extension)
1 cycle:	5 min	72°C (extension)
Final step:	Soak	4°C (hold)

4. Remove samples four at a time using a multichannel pipettor and apply directly to 1.5% agarose gels (e.g., 20×20 cm, Pharmacia Biotech) containing three or four rows of 22 lanes.

The primers used in this amplification protocol anneal to sites in the pCRII vector that are approximately 100 bp on each side of the cloning site. Colonies that contain plasmids with no inserts give a fragment of 205 bp, and colonies that contain plasmids with inserts give bands of 205 bp plus the size of the insert. Given that multiple cDNA species of the same size can be amplified from the same differential display band, 6 to 12 colonies from each ligation should be screened. At least two to four colonies that produce fragments of the correct size should be selected and subsequently screened for differential expression.

Differential Display PCR 113

D. Confirmation of Altered Expression by Dot-Blot Differential Hybridization

The confirmation of differentially expressed genes is the most time-consuming aspect of DD PCR. In the following method a dot-blot manifold is utilized whereby 96 clones may be examined simultaneously. Two membranes will be prepared, one for each treatment group to be examined. Control genes should be included in the differential hybridization screen to determine the success of the screen. At least one gene that is not expected to change after treatment (a loading control) and a gene that is expected to change after treatment in a defined manner should be included. This protocol can be easily modified to screen fragments with cDNAs from four tissues instead of two by increasing the amount of fragment amplified and distributing the fragments equally among four blots.

Protocol — Dot-Blot Differential Hybridization

1. Spot colonies to be screened onto a 150-mm master agar plate with appropriate selective media in the 96-well format and allow to grow overnight at 37°C.

2. With a multichannel pipettor, simultaneously touch 12 colonies in a row with 12 pipet tips. Eject tips containing the bacteria into PCR tubes containing 70 μL of amplification mix. Once the bacteria have been transferred, remove the tips, being careful not to contaminate neighboring tubes.

3. Amplify the fragments following the protocol in Colony-PCR.

4. Confirm amplification of the expected fragments by resolving 7 μL of each reaction on agarose gels as described above.

5. Transfer the remaining fragments into a 96-well microtiter plate.

6. Denature fragments by adding 7 μL of 3 M NaOH to each well. Mix by pipetting up and down. Incubate the plate (covered) at 65°C for 1 hr.

7. Neutralize the solution by adding 30 μL of 20X SSC. Mix well by pipetting up and down.

8. Pipet equal volumes (35 μL) of the DNA fragments (~100 to 500 μg) onto a prewashed nylon membrane (Hybond-N+, Amersham) via a 96-well dot-blot apparatus (e.g., Schleicher and Schull, Keene, NH) overlaid with 200 μL of 6X SSC to achieve even distribution of the fragment across the dot. Wash wells with 200 μL of 6X SSC. The DNA fragments are added to the dot-blot apparatus 4 rows at a time. The DNA fragments in rows A–D of the microtiter plate are added twice to one dot-blot 96-well array: once in rows A–D and once in rows E–H. The DNA fragments in rows E–H of the microtiter plate are then added twice to the next dot-blot 96-well array.

9. Take the membrane out of the dot-blot apparatus and mark the membrane to orient the dots. Wet the membrane in denaturing solution for 5 min.

114 PCR Protocols in Molecular Toxicology

10. Transfer the membrane to a filter paper wad soaked in neutralizing solution for 1 min.

11. Blot dry with filter paper. Air-dry or dry at 80°C for 10 min. Cut the membrane in half to separate the two halves containing the identical array of fragments.

12. Fix the DNA to the membrane. Wrap the membranes in Saran Wrap, place DNA-side down, and crosslink DNAs to the membrane with a transilluminator (e.g., StrataLinker, Stratagene).

13. Synthesize the cDNA from the treatment groups being compared. In each reaction, add:

    H_2O to 12 μL
    Total RNA (1 to 5 μg) or mRNA (50 to 500 ng)
    1 μL oligo(dT)$_{12-18}$ primer (500 μg/mL)

    Heat the mixture to 70°C for 10 min and quick-chill on ice. Collect the contents of the tube by brief centrifugation. Add:

    4 μL 5 × First-strand buffer
    2 μL 0.1 M DTT
    1 μL 10 mM dNTP mix

    Mix contents of the tube gently and incubate at 42°C for 2 min. Add 1 μL (200 U) of SuperScript II (Gibco-BRL) reverse transcriptase and mix by pipetting gently up and down. Incubate 50 min at 42°C. Inactivate the reaction by heating at 70°C for 15 min.

14. Label the cDNAs using the components of the Prime-It II random primer labeling kit (Stratagene) or other commercially available kit for labeling DNA. The probes should be at least 1×10^9 dpm/μg cDNA.

15. Prehybridize the membranes in prehybridization solution at 65°C for at least 1 h in a shaking water bath or in a rotary hybridization oven.

16. Add the labeled probes to the prehybridization solutions and incubate for at least 12 h at 65°C.

17. Wash filters by incubating in 2X SSC, 0.1% (w/v) SDS at room temperature for 10 min. Repeat.

18. Wash filters in 1X SSC, 0.1% SDS at 65°C for 15 min.

19. Wash filters in 0.2X SSC, 0.1% SDS at 65°C for 10 min.

20. Remove filters, wrap in Saran Wrap, and carry out autoradiography using intensifying screens at –80°C.

21. Develop X-ray film and compare the intensity of the spots between the two filters using the loading controls as measures of success of the experiment. The filters can be stripped of probe and then reprobed with different cDNAs from cells or individual genes.

Deviations from protocol. As an alternative to dot-blot differential hybridization, most groups have screened their fragments individually by

Differential Display PCR

Northern blot. A number of groups have increased the number of fragments that can be screened at one time by using slot-blot Northerns.[25,26] A technique called affinity capture has been used to isolate radioactively labeled cDNAs directly from Northern blots that hybridized to differentially expressed genes,[27] but this technique is labor-intensive and requires a large amount of RNA. Rapid grouping of the various cloned cDNAs found within one amplified band has been made using restriction enzymes that recognize 4 bp sequences[19] or by partial DNA sequencing and single-strand conformation analysis.[28] This analysis allows an informed selection of clones to screen. In addition, plasmids containing inserts have been subjected to dot-blot analysis using the original PCR-amplified DNA as a probe to confirm that the correct fragments have been cloned.[29] A T7 RNA polymerase binding site on the 5' end of the differential display fragment was incorporated so that riboprobes could be synthesized directly for subsequent ribonuclease protection assays.[30]

Reagents Needed

5X MMLV Buffer

250 mM Tris-HCl, pH 8.3
375 mM KCl
15 mM MgCl$_2$

10X Amplification Buffer

100 mM Tris-HCl, pH 8.4
500 mM KCl
15 mM MgCl$_2$
0.01% gelatin

Formamide Loading Buffer

95% formamide
0.09% w/v bromophenol blue
0.09% w/v xylene cyanol FF

6X Buffer

0.25% bromophenol blue
0.25% xylene cyanol FF
30% glycerol in H$_2$O

5X Ligation Buffer

0.25 M Tris-HCl (pH 7.6)
50 mM MgCl$_2$

PCR Protocols in Molecular Toxicology

50 m*M* dithiothreitol
250 µg/mL bovine serum albumin (Fraction V; Sigma) (optional)

Amplification Mix

200 µ*M* dNTPs
10 m*M* Tris, pH 8.3
1.5 m*M* $MgCl_2$
50 m*M* KCl
5% glycerol
0.1 µg/µL cresol red
0.6 U *Taq*
15 pmoles each of forward and reverse primers for amplification of inserts cloned into the polylinker of plasmid pCRII and most other cloning vectors encoding *lacZ'* (M13 forward, 5'-GTTTTCCCAGTCACGACGTTG-3' and M13 reverse, 5'-CAGGAAACAGCTATGACCATG-3')

Note: *The glycerol and cresol red are added to replace glycerol and bromophenol blue normally found in the 6X buffer.*

20X SSC

3 *M* NaCl
0.3 *M* sodium citrate

Prehybridization Solution

5X SSC
5X Denhardt's solution
0.5% (w/v) SDS
20 µg/mL of sonicated salmon sperm DNA, denatured by heating to 100°C for 5 min

100X Denhardt's Solution

2% (w/v) bovine serum albumin
2% (w/v) Ficoll™
2% (w/v) polyvinylpyrrolidone

Denaturing Solution

1.5 *M* NaCl
0.5 *M* NaOH

Differential Display PCR

Neutralizing Solution

> 1.5 *M* NaCl
> 0.5 *M* Tris-HCl, pH 7.2
> 0.001 *M* EDTA

5X First-Strand Buffer

> 250 m*M* Tris-HCl, pH 8.3
> 375 m*M* KCl
> 15 m*M* $MgCl_2$

Additional Reagents

Total cellular RNA or poly(A) RNA
1 U/μl human placental RNase inhibitor
10 U/μl DNase I (RNase-free)
3:1 (v/v) phenol/chloroform
3 *M* sodium acetate, pH 5.2
100%, 70%, and 85% ethanol
Diethylpyrocarbonate (DEPC)-treated H_2O
0.1 *M* dithiothreitol (DTT)
250 μ*M* and 25 μ*M* 4dNTP mixes
10 μ*M* each anchored oligo(dT) primer (e.g., Genehunter): 5′-T_{12}MG-3′, 5′-T_{12}MA-3′, 5′-T_{12}MG-3′, and 5′-T_{12}MC-3′ or set of 12 5′-T_{12}VN-3′ primers (where M represents dG, dA, and dC; N = dA, dC, dG, or dT; V = dA, dC, or dG)
200 U/μl Moloney murine leukemia virus (MoMuLV) reverse transcriptase
10 μCi/μl [α-^{35}S]dATP (>1200 Ci/mmol)
2 μ*M* arbitrary decamers (e.g., GeneHunter)
Taq DNA polymerase (5 U/μl)
Mineral oil
65°, 95°, 80°, and 100°C water baths
Thermal cycler
Whatman 3MM filter paper

References

1. **Wan, J.S., Sharp, S.J., Poirier, G.M.-C., Wagaman, P.C., Chambers, J., Pyati, J., Hom, Y.-L., Galindo, J.E., Huvar, A., Peterson, P.A., Jackson, M.R., and Erlander, M.G.,** Cloning differentially expressed mRNAs, *Nature Biotech.,* 14, 1685, 1996.
2. **Liang, P. and Pardee, A.B.,** Differential display of eukaryotic messenger RNA by means of the polymerase chain reaction, *Science,* 257, 967, 1992.

3. **McClellan, M., Mathieu-Daude, F., and Welsch, J.,** RNA fingerprinting and differential display using arbitrarily primed PCR, *Trends in Genetics*, 11, 242, 1995.

4. **Corton, J.C. and Gustafsson, J.-A.,** Increased efficiency in screening large numbers of cDNA fragments generated by differential display, *BioTechniques*, 22, 802, 1997.

5. **Zeiner, M. and Gehring, U.,** Cloning of 5′ cDNA regions by inverse PCR, *BioTechniques*, 17, 1051, 1994.

6. **Sompayrac, L., Jane, S., Burn, T.C., Tenen, D.G., and Danna, K.J.,** Overcoming limitations of the mRNA differential display technique, *Nucleic Acids Res.*, 23, 4738, 1995.

7. **Sokolov, B.P. and Prockop, D.J.,** A rapid and simple PCR-based method for isolation of cDNAs from differentially expressed genes, *Nucleic Acids Res.*, 22, 4009, 1994.

8. **Bertioli, D.J., Schlichter, U.H.A., Adams, M.J., Burrows, P.R., Steinbiß, H.-H., and Antoniw, J.F.,** An analysis of differential display shows a strong bias towards high copy number mRNAs, *Nucleic Acids Res.*, 23, 4520, 1995.

9. **Guimarães, M.J., Lee, F., Ziotnik, A., and McClanahan, T.,** Differential display by PCR: novel findings and applications, *Nucleic Acids Res.*, 23, 1832, 1995.

10. **Ausubel, F.M., Brent, R., Kingston, R.E., Moore, D.D., Seidman, J.G., Smith, J.A., and Struhl, K.,** *Current Protocols in Molecular Biology*, Green Publishing Associates and Wiley-Interscience, 1988.

11. **Chomczynski, P. and Sacchi, N.,** Single step method for RNA isolation by acid guanidinium-thiocyanate-phenol-chloroform extraction, *Anal. Biochem.*, 162, 156, 1987.

12. **Bauer, D., Muller, H., Reich, J., Riedel, H., Ahrenkiel, V., Warthoe, P., and Strauss, M.,** Identification of differentially expressed mRNA species by an improved display technique (DDRT-PCR), *Nucleic Acids Res.*, 21, 4272, 1993.

13. **Liang, P., Averboukh, L., and Pardee, A.B.,** Distribution and cloning of eukaryotic mRNAs by means of differential display: refinements and optimization, *Nucleic Acids Res.*, 21, 3269, 1993.

14. **Liang, P. Bauer, D, Averboukh, L, Warthoe, P, Rohrwild, M, Muller, H, Strauss, M, and Pardee, A.B.** Analysis of altered gene expression by differential display, *Methods in Enzymology*, 254, 304, 1995.

15. **Adatti, N., Ito, T., Koga, C., Kito, K., Sakaki, Y., and Shiokawa, K.,** Differential display analysis of gene expression in developing embryos of Xenopus laevis, *Biochim. Biophys. Acta*, 1262, 43, 1995.

16. **Chen, J.J.W. and Peck, K.,** Non-radioisotopic differential display method to directly visualize and amplify differential bands on nylon membrane, *Nucleic Acids Res.*, 24, 793, 1996.

17. **Lohmann, J., Schickle, H., and Bosch, T.C.G.,** REN display, a rapid and efficient method for nonradioactive differential display and mRNA isolation, *BioTechniques*, 18, 200, 1995.

Differential Display PCR

18. **Linskens, M.H.K., Feng, J., Andres, W.H., Enlow, B.E., Saati, S.M., Tonkin, L.A., Funk, W.D., and Villeponteau, B.,** Cataloging altered gene expression in young and senescent cells using enhanced differential display, *Nucleic Acids Res.*, 23, 3244, 1995.

19. **Shoham, N.G., Arad, T., Rosin-Abersfeld, R., Mashian, P., Gazit, A., and Yaniv, A.,** Differential display assay and analysis, *BioTechniques*, 20, 182, 1996.

20. **Diachenko, L.B., Ledesma, J., Chenchik, A.A., and Siebert, P.D.,** Combining the technique of RNA fingerprinting and differential display to obtain differentially expressed mRNA, *Biochem. Biophys. Res. Commun.*, 219, 824-, 1996.

21. **Yoshikawa, T., Xing, G., and Detera-Wadleigh, S.D.,** Detection, simultaneous display and direct sequencing of multiple nuclear hormone receptor genes using bilaterally targeted RNA fingerprinting, *Biochim et Biophys Acta*, 1264, 63, 1995.

22. **Johnson, S.W., Lissy, N.A., Miller, P.D., Testa, J.R., Ozols, R.F., and Hamilton, T.C.,** Identification of zinc finger mRNAs using domain-specific differential display, *Anal. Biochem.*, 236, 348, 1996.

23. **Suzuki, Y., Sato, N., Tohyama, M., Wanaka, A., and Takagi, T.,** Efficient isolation of differentially expressed genes by means of a newly established method, 'ESD,' *Nucleic Acids Res.*, 24, 797, 1996.

24. **Gussow, D. and Clackson, T.,** Direct clone characterization from plaques and colonies by the polymerase chain reaction, *Nucleic Acids Res.*, 17, 4000, 1989.

25. **Corton, J.C., Bocos, C., Moreno, E.S., Merritt, A., Marsman, D.S., Sausen, P.J., Cattley, R.C., and Gustafsson, J.-A.,** The rat 17β-estradiol dehydrogenase is a novel peroxisome-proliferator-inducible gene, *Molec. Pharmacol.*, 50, 1157, 1996.

26. **Vögeli-Lange, R., Bürckert, N., Boller, T., and Wiemken, A.,** Rapid selection and classification of positive clones generated by mRNA differential display, *Nucleic Acids Res.*, 24, 1385, 1996.

27. **Li, F, Barnathan, E.S. and Karikó, K.,** Rapid method for screening and cloning cDNAs generated in differential mRNA display: application of northern blot for affinity capturing of cDNA. *Nucleic Acids Res.*, 22, 1764. 1994.

28. **Zhao, S., Ooi, S.L., Yang, F.-C., and Pardee, A.B.,** Three methods for identification of true positive cloned cDNA fragments in differential display, *BioTechniques*, 20, 400, 1996.

29. **Callard, D., Lescure, B., and Mazzolini, L.,** A method for the elimination of false positives generated by the mRNA differential display technique, *BioTechniques*, 16, 1096, 1994.

30. **Yeatman, T.J. and Mao, W.,** Identification of a differentially-expressed message associated with colon cancer liver metastasis using an improved method of differential display, *Nucleic Acids Res.*, 23, 4007, 1995.

Chapter 4

Cloning by PCR

John. P. Vanden Heuvel

Contents

I.	Introduction	122
II.	Basic TA Cloning	122
	A. Basic Considerations	122
	B. Construction of TA Cloning Vector	123
	C. Ligation of PCR Product	125
III.	Basic Cloning by RT–PCR	126
	A. Basic Considerations	126
	Protocol	127
IV.	Degenerate Primer PCR	131
	Protocol	133
V.	RACE: Rapid Amplification of cDNA Ends	134
	A. Amplification of cDNA 3′ Ends	135
	B. Amplification of cDNA 5′ Ends	137
VI.	Library Screening by PCR	139
	Protocol 1: Dilution Screening	140
	Protocol 2: Enrichment Screening by PCR	142
	Protocol 3: Library RACE	144
VII.	Examination of DNA-Protein Interactions. Selection and Binding Sites (SAAB) Technique	145
	A. General Considerations	145
	Protocol	147
	DNA Binding Site Library Synthesis	147
	First Round Selection (Gel Shift Assay)	148
	Electrophoresis of DNA-Protein Complexes	148
	Amplification of Selected DNA Pool	149

0-8493-3344-X/98/$0.00+$.50
© 1998 by CRC Press LLC

	Subsequent Rounds of Selection	150
VIII.	PCR Clone Check	152
	Protocol	152
IX.	Direct Sequencing by PCR	154
	Protocol	154
Reagents Needed		155
References		160

I.   Introduction

Since its advent, PCR has revolutionized how genes are cloned, decreasing the time required to obtain a clone and making the process technically less challenging. The following chapter will highlight several sets of methods that can utilize PCR for cloning; each is based on the amount of information one has on the target gene. First, the ability to add DNA sequences on the 5′ end of primers has made subcloning much simpler, especially when unique restriction enzyme sites within the gene and plasmid are difficult to find. The unique feature of *Taq* polymerase adding a single 3′-A overhang makes PCR cloning into T-overhang vectors an efficient alternative to the use of restriction endonucleases. Second, since the stringency of PCR is easily controlled by conditions such as Mg^{2+} concentration, annealing time and temperature, degenerate nucleotides, and PCR additives, cloning genes based on similarity has become a slightly less daunting task. This is especially true when trying to clone low expression genes or genes from tissues where a library is not readily obtainable. Third, the identification of sequences surrounding a known sequence can be found much more rapidly using PCR than if library screening was used. Several complementary PCR techniques can be used to identify flanking sequences, including rapid amplification of cDNA ends (RACE), anchored PCR, and PCR library screening. The fourth section will discuss a procedure that will identify sequences recognized by DNA binding proteins. This method is used to clone sequences recognized by transcription factors and regulatory proteins that interact with specific sequences of DNA. Several basic PCR procedures that are used in most of these methods will also be discussed. These include clone checking and sequencing procedures that utilize PCR techniques.

II.   Basic TA Cloning

2.   Basic Considerations

The basic concept of PCR, or TA, cloning has been discussed to some extent in Chapter 2 in the context of internal standard synthesis. The premise of TA cloning is that certain thermostable polymerases add a single deoxyadenosine

Cloning by PCR

TABLE 4.1

Comparison of Thermostable DNA Polymerases

Characteristic	Taq	Tth	Vent	Deep Vent	Pfu
Type of end generated upon PCR amplification	3'A	3'A	>95% Blunt	>95% Blunt	Blunt
5' to 3' exonuclease activity	Yes	Yes	No	No	No
3' to 5' exonuclease activity	No	No	Yes	Yes	Yes

to the 3' end of amplified fragments in a template-independent fashion. A vector is either purchased or produced which contains a complementary T overhang at the insertion point. Ligation of the PCR product into such a vector is more efficient than blunt-end cloning, but much less efficient than sticky-end (produced by restriction endonucleases, discussed in the subsequent section). An important choice one must make when implementing a PCR cloning project is which thermostable DNA polymerase to use. The lack of a 3'-A overhang will preclude TA cloning. Also, 3' to 5' exonuclease activity may be desirable to increase "proof-reading" and decrease the chances of introducing a PCR-related mutation (see a summary in Table 4.1). Of course, when changing enzymes, one must also re-optimize the PCR reaction including the buffer system, $MgCl_2$, annealing temperature, and nucleotide concentration.

B. Construction of TA Cloning Vector

For a review of cloning vectors, see references 1 and 2.

Protocol

1. Choose a plasmid vector that contains a unique, blunt-end cutting restriction enzyme site such as SmaI or EcoRV. Set up the following digestion reaction:

Note: *The vector used to clone PCR products may be a critical consideration. Several commercially available vectors have shown problems including high background, low copy number, and instability of T-ends.[3] It may be advisable to avoid unnecessarily large cloning regions to reduce the risk of unstable vectors.*

ddH$_2$O	up to 20 µl
10X restriction enzyme buffer (supplied with enzyme)	2 µl
Cloning vector	5 µg
Blunt-end enzyme	10 units

124　　　　　　　　　　　　　　　　　　　PCR Protocols in Molecular Toxicology

2. Allow the digestion to proceed at 37°C for at least three hours. Heat inactivate the enzyme at 65°C for 15 min.

3. Add 20 μl (1 volume) TE-buffered phenol/chloroform (1:1, v/v), vortex for 1 min, and centrifuge for 2 min at 12,000 × g.

4. Carefully remove the top, aqueous layer and transfer to a fresh tube. Add 10 μl (0.5 volume) 7.5 M ammonium acetate and 40 μl (2 volumes) chilled 100% ethanol. Vortex briefly and precipitate at –70°C for 30 min.

5. Centrifuge at 12,000 × g for 10 minutes, decant the supernatant, and briefly rinse the pellet with 1 ml 70% ethanol. Dry the pellet for 15 min under vacuum and dissolve the linearized plasmid in 15 μl ddH$_2$O.

6. Take 2 μl of the sample to measure the concentration of the DNA using UV spectroscopy. Estimate the amount of DNA present using the following formula:

$$\mu g/\mu l \text{ sample} = \text{Absorption at 260 nm} \times 0.04 \ \mu g/\mu l \times \text{dilution factor}$$

7. Since circularized, uncut plasmid can cause very high background in subsequent experiments, care must be taken to assure that only the cut, linearized plasmid is present. Take a 2 μl aliquot and resolve on an 0.8% agarose gel. If complete digestion did not occur, repeat Steps 1 through 6.

8. This plasmid can now be used to generate a T-overhang vector. Set up the following PCR reaction in the order listed, enough for five reactions.

Component	μl	Final Concentration
ddH$_2$O	171	—
MgCl$_2$ (25 mM)	40	3 mM
10X buffer	25	1X
dTTP (100 mM)	1.2	0.4 mM
Linearized plasmid	10	up to 1 μg/tube
Taq DNA polymerase (5 U/μl)	2	2 units/tube

9. Pipet 50 μl into each of four tubes. Incubate at 72°C for 1 h. Pool the four reactions.

10. Add 200 μl (1 volume) TE-buffered phenol/chloroform (1:1, v/v), vortex for 1 min, and centrifuge for 2 min at 12,000 × g.

11. Carefully remove the top, aqueous layer and transfer to a fresh tube. Add 100 μl (0.5 volume) 7.5 M ammonium acetate and 400 μl (2 volumes) chilled 100% ethanol. Vortex briefly and precipitate at –70°C for 30 min.

12. Centrifuge at 12,000 × g for 10 min, decant the supernatant, and briefly rinse the pellet with 1 ml 70% ethanol. Dry the pellet for 15 min under vacuum and dissolve the linearized plasmid in 50 μl ddH$_2$O.

13. Take 2 μl of the sample to measure the concentration of the DNA using UV spectroscopy. Estimate the amount of DNA present using the following formula:

Cloning by PCR

$\mu g/\mu l$ sample = Absorption at 260 nm × 0.04 $\mu g/\mu l$ × dilution factor

C. Ligation of PCR Product

1. Pool and purify PCR products as stated previously. Analyze PCR products on an agarose gel.
2. Set up the following ligation reactions, on ice.

Ligation Reaction

ddH$_2$O	up to 20 μl
10X Ligation buffer	2
Linearized plasmid	100 ng
PCR product	400 ng
T4 DNA ligase	10 units

Control Ligation Reaction

ddH$_2$O	up to 20 μl
10X Ligation buffer	2
Linearized plasmid	100 ng
PCR product	0
T4 DNA ligase	10 units

3. Incubate at 15°C overnight. Stop the reaction at 70°C for 10 min.

Note: *If a high background is obtained (i.e., a large amount of self-ligated vector), it may be advantageous to repeat the ligation reaction at 4°C overnight. This will decrease the overall yield of clones, but may increase the specificity of the ligation reaction (higher percentage of positive clones).*

4. For heat-shock transformation of *E. coli* follow the procedures listed below. Each bacterial strain has different optimal transformation conditions. The appropriate conditions for DH5α cells (Gibco BRL), a good, standard efficiency strain that allows for blue-white screening, are given.

   i. Thaw competent *E. coli* on ice

   ii. Add 10 μl ligation reaction to 50 μl *E. coli* and let sit on ice for 30 min

   iii. Place in 37°C water for 30 sec

   iv. Put tubes back on ice for 2 min

126 PCR Protocols in Molecular Toxicology

    v. Add 1 mL LB or SOC media

    vi. Shake tubes (220 rpm) at 37°C for 1 h

    vii. Spin briefly in a microfuge, remove supernatant, and *gently* resuspend in 100 µl LB media

    viii. Spread 90 µl and 10 µl on each of two LB agar plates (with IPTG and X-Gal if blue-white screening is performed)

    ix. Grow inverted at 37°C overnight

5. Check colonies for the presence of inserts as discussed in a subsequent section (PCR clone check).

III.   Basic Cloning by RT–PCR

A.   Basic Considerations

The following RT–PCR procedure is a relatively simple, rapid, and inexpensive method to clone a gene of interest. The only criteria required for this method is that the sequence of the mRNA or DNA be known. (A case where the sequence is not fully known is discussed subsequently.) Primers are chosen that will amplify the area of interest within the gene (i.e., full coding sequence, putative DNA binding domain, etc.). The real strength of utilizing PCR to subclone DNA fragments is the fact that recombinant DNA can be easily formed. That is, the primers may be designed such that the 3′ end will recognize the target gene, while the 5′ end can contain restriction enzyme sites. A similar method was discussed in Chapter 2, where a recombinant DNA molecule with an RNA polymerase site was constructed. Virtually any sequence may be added to the primers, including translation start and stop sites, antibody recognition sequences (epitopes), hybridization sequences for Southern blots, nested primer sites, and polyadenylation signals. The only possible limitations may be the length of the primers used (there is a decrease in amplification efficiency with long primers, i.e., >40mer), and the fact that artifacts of PCR may be difficult to avoid.[4]

The basic design of the primers used to clone a gene are as follows:[5]

Cloning forward primer: 5′ Clamp — Restriction enzyme site 1 — gene-specific forward primer 3′

Cloning reverse primer: 5′ Clamp — Restriction enzyme site 2 — gene-specific reverse primer 3′

The salient features of the primers include (5′ to 3′) the clamp sequence, the restriction enzyme site, and 18 to 24 bases of gene-specific bases. The clamp sequence is two to five bases of arbitrary sequence to aid in the subsequent endonuclease digestion, such as ATA- or GC-. Consult the supplier of the

Cloning by PCR

enzyme for information on whether it is an efficient "end cutter" and if the clamp sequence needs to be lengthened. The restriction enzyme sequences should not be contained within the DNA segment to be cloned but must be within the cloning site of the appropriate vector. If the direction of the insert is important (i.e., placing a gene under control of a promoter contained on the vector), the restriction enzyme site 1 and 2 should be different. If the insert can go in the plasmid in either direction, the enzyme site on the primers may be the same. The gene-specific primers may be tested prior to the inclusion of the 5′ extra sequences. Care must be taken with reverse primer design to ensure that the reverse complement (i.e., the sequence that would result on the top, coding or + strand) will result in the proper sequence.

Protocol

1. Extract total RNA or poly(A)+RNA from the tissue of interest. See Chapter 6 for details on extraction procedures.

2. Design the primers needed to amplify the region of interest. See the considerations above and reference 6 for primer design.

Note: *Several restriction endonuclease sites have proven to be difficult to incorporate effectively into the PCR product. Sites such as NotI, XhoI, and XbaI incorporated into the termini of PCR products do not cut efficiently.[6] If these enzymes cannot be avoided, the length of the clamp may require optimization.*

3. Prepare the following for the first-strand cDNA synthesis and place on ice. The recipe is enough for 10 tubes. (The final reaction volume will be 20 µl).

Note: *It is advisable to perform multiple tubes of RT–PCR instead of using high cycle number to obtain a sufficient amount of DNA for cloning. Although the error rate of Taq is relatively low, there is always a risk of incurring a mutation when running too many cycles.*

Component	µl	*Final Concentration*
ddH$_2$O	116	—
MgCl$_2$ (25 mM)	36	5 mM
10X PCR buffer	18	1X
dATP (100 mM)	1.8	1 mM
dCTP (100 mM)	1.8	1 mM
dGTP (100 mM)	1.8	1 mM

PCR Protocols in Molecular Toxicology

dTTP (100 mM)	1.8	1 mM
Oligo(dT)$_{15}$ (0.5 mg/ml)*	2.3	6 µg/ml
rRNasin (30 U/µl)	2.3	7.5 U
Total RNA (0.05 µg/µl)	16	100 ng/tube

* Random hexamers may be substituted for Oligo(dT)$_{15}$.
Also, if a low expression gene is to be cloned, the reverse
primer (without the clamp and restriction enzyme sites)
may be used.

4. Add 2.5 µl (500 U) MMLV reverse transcriptase to the cDNA mixture. Vortex briefly.

Note: *MMLV is the most common type of reverse transcriptase used in cDNA synthesis. AMV reverse transcriptase may be substituted, but use 5 units/tube. If the cDNA to be cloned is a relatively long sequence, specialty grade reverse transcriptase (i.e., Superscript II, Gibco BRL) may be substituted. Follow the manufacturer's suggestions for cDNA synthesis conditions.*

5. Add 20 µl cDNA mix to the PCR tubes. Cap tubes and vortex briefly to mix.
6. Place in the thermocycler and run the following program:

42°C for 30 min
95°C for 5 min
Store at 4°C

7. While the cDNA synthesis is proceeding, assemble the PCR mixture as follows, at room temperature.

Component	µl	Final Concentration (in PCR reaction)*
ddH$_2$O	20 0	—
MgCl$_2$ (25 mM)	36	4 mM
10X PCR buffer	27	1X
Cloning forward primer (10 pmol/µl)	27	30 pmol
Cloning reverse primer (10 pmol/µl)	27	30 pmol

* The cDNA reaction contains nucleotides, additional MgCl$_2$, and 10X buffer. The final concentration of nucleotides is 400 µM.

Cloning by PCR

8. When the cDNA reaction is complete, choose one of two methods for assembly of the PCR reaction: hot start (Steps 9 through 12) or cold start (Steps 13 through 15).

Note: *Two different methods can be used in an attempt to decrease mispriming and primer artifacts and to ensure that all the tubes will start amplification simultaneously. In a hot start all the reagents (cDNA reactions, PCR master mix) are brought to 85°C prior to the addition of Taq. This will prevent the primers from binding to each other and will also dissociate the primers from the template. The easiest way to perform a hot start is to use a heat block that will hold the standard PCR tube. In a cold start the cDNA and the PCR mix are placed on ice. This method is technically easier and there is less chance of contamination, but the efficiency of amplification is much less than when using a hot start.*

Hot Start

9. Immediately prior to completion of the cDNA reaction, place the mix prepared in Step 7 in an 85°C heat block (3 to 5 min).

10. At the completion of the cDNA reaction, remove the tubes from the thermocycler and place them in an 85°C heat block. (The thermocycler may also be used as a surrogate heat block.) Add 2.5 μl *Taq* DNA polymerase (5 U/μl) to the preheated mix. Vortex and return to the heat block.

11. Add 30 μl PCR mix directly to the tube containing the cDNA reaction in the heat block. Work quickly to avoid evaporation.

12. Place the reactions in the thermocycler only when it has reached at least 85°C. A sample PCR reaction is given below. The temperature, times, and cycles must be optimized for each primer pair.

Denature	94°C 4 min
	<u>Cycle (26X)</u>
Denature	94°C 20 sec
Anneal	60°C 30 sec
Elongate	72°C 30 sec
Elongate	72°C 5 min
Store	4°C

Cold Start

13. Prepare the PCR mix as suggested in Step 7. Place on ice.

130   PCR Protocols in Molecular Toxicology

14. At the completion of the cDNA reaction, remove the tubes from the thermocycler and place them on ice. Add 2.5 µl *Taq* DNA polymerase (5 U/µl) to the cold mix. Vortex and place back on ice.

15. Add 30 µl PCR mix directly to the tube containing the cDNA reaction on ice.

16. Place the reactions in the thermocycler and run the optimized PCR program.

17. Pool the PCR products and chloroform/phenol extract (see Chapter 6). Dissolve the pellet in 25 µl ddH$_2$O. Resolve 2 µl on an agarose and quantitate 5 µl by spectrophotometry.

Ligation Reaction

1. Digest the plasmid vector and the PCR product with the appropriate restriction enzymes.

ddH$_2$O	up to 20 µl
10X restriction enzyme buffer (supplied with enzyme)	2 µl
Vector or PCR product	2.5 µg
Restriction enzyme	10 units

2. Allow the digestion to proceed at 37°C for at least three hours. Heat inactivate the enzyme at 65°C for 15 minutes.

3. Set the tube containing the restriction enzyme digestion for the PCR product on ice. To the vector digestion add 2.2 µl 10X alkaline phosphatase buffer and 1 µl (3 units) calf intestinal alkaline phosphatase. Incubate at 37°C for 15 min and 5 min at 65°C.

4. Add 20 µl (1 volume) TE-buffered phenol/chloroform (1:1, v/v) to each tube, vortex for 1 min and centrifuge for 2 min at 12,000 × *g*.

5. Carefully remove the top, aqueous layer and transfer to a fresh tube. Add 10 µl (0.5 volume) 7.5 *M* ammonium acetate and 40 µl (2 volumes) chilled 100% ethanol. Vortex briefly and precipitate at –70°C for 30 min.

6. Centrifuge at 12,000 × *g* for 10 min, decant the supernatant, and briefly rinse the pellet with 1 ml 70% ethanol. Dry the pellet for 15 min under vacuum and dissolve both products in 15 µl ddH$_2$O.

7. Take 2 µl of the sample to measure the concentration of the DNA using UV spectroscopy. Estimate the amount of DNA present using the following formula:

$$\mu g/\mu l \text{ sample} = \text{Absorption at 260 nm} \times 0.04\ \mu g/\mu l \times \text{dilution factor}$$

8. Since circularized, uncut plasmid can cause very high background in subsequent experiments, care must be taken to assure that only the cut, linearized plasmid is present. Take a 2 µl aliquot and resolve on a 0.8% agarose gel. If complete digestion did not occur, repeat Steps 1 through 7.

9. Construct the following ligation reactions, on ice:

Cloning by PCR

Ligation Reaction

ddH$_2$O	up to 20 μl
10X Ligation buffer	2
Linearized plasmid	100 ng
PCR product	400 ng
T4 DNA ligase	10 units

Control Ligation Reaction

ddH$_2$O	up to 20 μl
10X Ligation buffer	2
Linearized plasmid	100 ng
PCR product	0
T4 DNA ligase	10 units

10. Incubate at 15°C overnight. Stop the reaction at 70°C for 10 min.

11. For heat-shock transformation of *E. coli* follow the procedures listed below. Each bacterial strain has different optimal transformation conditions. The appropriate conditions for DH5α cells (Gibco BRL), a good, standard efficiency strain that allows for blue-white screening, are given.

  i.   Thaw competent *E. coli* on ice

  ii. Add 10 μl ligation reaction to 50 μl *E. coli* and let sit on ice for 30 min

  iii. Place in 37°C water for 30 sec

  iv. Put tubes back on ice for 2 minutes

  v.   Add 1 mL LB or SOC media (See Chapter 6)

  vi. Shake tubes (220 rpm) at 37°C for 1 h

  vii. Spin briefly in a microfuge, remove supernatant, and *gently* resuspend in 100 μl LB media

  viii. Spread 90 μl and 10 μl on each of two LB agar plates (with IPTG and X-Gal if blue-white screening is performed) containing the appropriate antibiotic.

  ix. Grow inverted at 37°C overnight

12. Check colonies for the presence of inserts as discussed subsequently.

IV.   Degenerate Primer PCR

Often when a cDNA is cloned, it is of interest to determine whether related genes exist. This can be done using several approaches which include screening

TABLE 4.2
Degeneracy of the Amino Acid Codons

Amino Acid	Codons
L,R,S	6
A,G,P,T,V	4
I	3
C,D,E,F,H,K,N,Q,Y	2
M,W	1

expression libraries with cross-reacting antibodies or cDNA libraries with low stringency hybridization or PCR techniques. In the following example, degenerate primers are used to amplify regions of a gene that are conserved at the protein or amino acid levels. In addition, this type of primer may be used when only amino acid sequences are known and cDNA sequences are sought. Degenerate primers contain mixtures of oligonucleotides or a nonspecific nucleotide (i.e., one that will base-pair with more than one other nucleotide). Degenerate oligonucleotides are useful when only the protein sequence is known or when the goal is to amplify many members of a family of proteins for subsequent identification.

A critical factor in designing degenerative primers is the redundancy of the genetic code.[7] As shown in Table 4.2, several codons may be used for a single amino acid, such as six codons for lycine, arginine, and serine. Methionine and tryptophan are encoded by a single codon. It is critical that the primers used have a minimal amount of degeneracy. Therefore, if possible, the amino acids with four or six codons should be avoided. When evaluating several peptide sequences for subsequent primer design, one should add the possible number of codons given in Table 4.2 and try to choose from the area with the lowest degeneracy. Other critical considerations are[7]: 1) avoid a primer with a 3′ degenerative base; 2) shorter primers (15 to 18 bp) are preferred because of the decreased degeneracy and increased specificity; and 3) since codon bias is often seen (i.e., not all four codons of arginine are used in mammalian species), the degenerative primer may be further restricted.

The last consideration when using degenerative primers is the choice of nucleotide. When the primer is synthesized, it can incorporate a mixture of nucleotides (i.e., R can be a G or an A) or a nucleotide that can base-pair with A, C, G, or T (i.e., inosine). Ambiguous nucleotides can be incorporated during the synthesis of the primers. Please consult Table 4.3 for the standard International Union of Biochemistry (IUB) code to use when ordering this type of primer. If a primer is highly degenerate, for example, it has many ambiguous bases, the mixture is very complex. That is, only a small subpopulation of the primer will be effective in amplifying the product of interest. On the other hand, inosine-containing primers are far less complex because they are not mixtures of different sequences. However, the strength of the inosine-contain-

Cloning by PCR

133

TABLE 4.3
Ambiguous DNA Codes
(International Union of Biochemistry)

G Guanosine	R = G or A puRine
A Adenosine	Y = C or T pYrimidine
T Thymidine	W = A or T Weak (2 H-bonds)
C Cytidine	S = C or G Strong (3 H-bonds)
	K = G or T Keto
	M = A or C aMino

B = C, G or T not A
D = A, G or T not C   N = A, C, G or T aNy
H = A, C or T not G   X = A, C, G or T
V = A, C or G not T

complementary	G A T C R Y W S K M B D H V N X
DNA	I I I I I I I I I I I I I I I I
strands	C T A G Y R W S M K V H D B N X

ing bonds is relatively weak compared to G-C base-pairing. This will result in the requirement of lower annealing temperatures and possibly decreased specificity of amplification. Also, inosine-containing primers are slightly more expensive than normal nucleotides. Our laboratory has had much more success with inosine-containing bases than the mixed nucleotides, and we see much more specific product at higher yield with the former.

Once designed, degenerate primers are very versatile and may be used in almost any PCR protocol. It is beyond the scope of the present chapter to go into great detail about all the uses of these primers. Suffice it to say that degenerate primers have been used in cDNA cloning, RACE, and library screening. For specific examples, see references 8, 9, 10, 11, and 12.

Protocol

1. Synthesize the appropriate degenerative primers, keeping in mind the criteria stated above.

2. With the degenerative primer, perform the PCR experiments as described in this chapter for traditional primers (i.e., RT–PCR cloning, library screening, and RACE). The optimization of the PCR must be rigorously examined.

Note: *Degenerative primers have been used extensively in RT–PCR and TA cloning, library screening, and various RACE techniques. Often, the degenerative or mixed primers will result in very specific amplification products. If this is the case, one could use these primers in quantitative or semiquantitative assays. However, it would be advisable to clone the product derived from the degenerative PCR and choose traditional primers from the internal sequence.*

3. Clone and sequence the degenerative PCR product as discussed in other sections of this book.

V. RACE: Rapid Amplification of cDNA Ends

Often when cloning a gene, be it by differential display (Chapter 3), library screening, or degenerate primer PCR, only a partial sequence is obtained. In this section, we will discuss a PCR-based method that can be used to obtain new information on the 5' and 3' end of the known cDNA sequence. This method has been termed rapid amplification of cDNA ends (RACE) and differs from library screening and other methods to obtain full-length sequences in that it may be performed in a relatively short period of time (two to three days).

The basic 5' and 3' RACE protocols are shown in Figure 4.1 and are based largely on the method of M.A. Frohman (reviewed in reference 13). Briefly, in 5' RACE, a gene-specific primer (GSP) is used to prime the reverse transcription reaction. Using terminal transferase, a homopolymer (poly A or polyT) is appended to the first-strand cDNA. Subsequently, PCR is used to amplify the region between the GSP and the homopolymer using the oligo dT

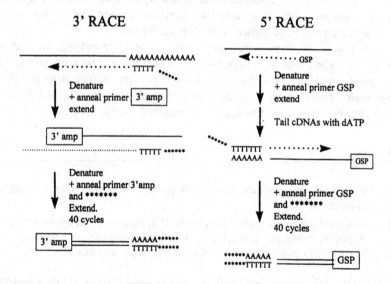

Figure 4.1
Basic procedures of 3' and 5' RACE. To perform 3' RACE (left panel), the oligo dT adapter primer is used in the reverse transcription reaction. This step adds a recognition site for the adapter primer on the 3' end of cDNA. In the PCR reaction, this adapter primer and the gene-specific forward primer are used to amplify the unknown region. In 5' RACE (right panel) a gene-specific primer (GSP) is used to prime the reverse transcription reaction. Using terminal transferase, a homopolymer (polyA or polyT) is appended to the first-strand cDNA. Subsequently, PCR is used to amplify the region between the GSP and the homopolymer using the oligo dT adapter primer and the gene specific primer. *** denotes the adapter sequence.

Cloning by PCR

adapter primer and the gene-specific primer. To perform 3' RACE, the oligo dT adapter primer is used in the reverse transcription reaction. This step adds a recognition site for the adapter primer on the 3' end of cDNA. In the PCR reaction this adapter primer and the gene-specific forward primer are used to amplify the unknown region.

The following sequences for the oligo dT adapter primer and adapter primer may be used,[13] although virtually any sequence may be incorporated. Gene-specific primers are designed using the suggestions in Chapter 1, or may be degenerate primers as discussed above.

Oligo dT adapter primer

GACTCGAGTCGACATCGATTTTTTTTTTTTTTTTT

Adapter primer

GACTCGAGTCGACATCGA

A. Amplification of cDNA 3' Ends

Protocol

Reverse Transcription

1. Prepare the following on ice.

Component	μl	Final Concentration
MgCl$_2$ (25 mM)	4	5 mM
10X PCR buffer	2	1X
dATP (10 mM)	1	1mM
dCTP (10 mM)	1	1mM
dGTP (10 mM)	1	1mM
dTTP (10 mM)	1	1mM
Oligo(dT)$_{17}$-adapter primer (0.5 mg/ml)	1	25 μg/ml
rRNasin (30 U/μl)	0.5	15 U
MMLV reverse transcriptase	0.5	100 U

2. Heat RNA in 8 μl of H$_2$O for 3 min at 65°C; quench on ice and add to the above. The final volume of the cDNA reaction is now 20 μl.

136 PCR Protocols in Molecular Toxicology

3. Incubate at 42°C for 1 hour and then at 52°C for 30 min. Dilute to 1 ml with TE and store at 4°C (cDNA pool).

PCR Amplification

1. Prepare the PCR mix.

Note: *DMSO has been reported to aid in reducing the secondary structure of DNA. This is particularly useful when trying to amplify regions with a high G:C content. This supplement may be removed and replaced with an additional 5 μl of ddH$_2$O*

Component	μl	Final Concentration
ddH$_2$O	25–30	up to 50 μl
10 X PCR buffer	5	1X
DMSO	5	10%
dATP (100 mM)	0.75	1.5 mM
dCTP (100 mM)	0.75	1.5 mM
dGTP (100 mM)	0.75	1.5 mM
dTTP (100 mM)	0.75	1.5 mM
Adapter primer (10 pmol/μl)	3μl	30 pmol
Gene-specific forward primer	3 μl	30 pmol
cDNA pool	1–5	

2. Denature PCR mix at 85°C for 3 to 5 min. Add 2.5 units of *Taq* polymerase (0.5 μl/tube).

3. Place the reactions in the thermocycler only when it has reached at least 85°C. A sample PCR reaction is given below. The temperature, times, and cycles may need to be optimized for each primer pair.

Cycle (1X)

Denature	94°C 4 min
Anneal	55°C 5 min
Elongate	72°C 30 min

Cloning by PCR

	Cycle (30X)
Denature	94°C 20 sec
Anneal	55°C 30 sec
Elongate	72°C 2 min
Elongate	72°C 5 min
Store	4°C

B.   Amplification of cDNA 5′ Ends

Protocol

Reverse Transcription

1. Prepare the following on ice. (Essentially identical to that stated above, except substitute 10 pmol gene-specific primer for oligo dT adapter primer.) Perform reverse transcription as shown above.

Component	μl	Final Concentration
MgCl$_2$ (25 mM)	4	5 mM
10X PCR buffer	2	1X
dATP (10 mM)	1	1 mM
dCTP (10 mM)	1	1 mM
dGTP (10 mM)	1	1 mM
dTTP (10 mM)	1	1 mM
Gene-specific reverse primer (0.5 mg/ml)	1	25 μg/ml
rRNasin (30 U/μl)	0.5	15 U
MMLV reverse transcriptase	0.5	100 U
RNA	8	100–1000 ng

2. Remove excess primer using any one of several purification methods (Centricon 100 spin filters, Wizard PCR Preps etc.). Concentrate to 10 μl using either vacuum centrifugation or ethanol precipitation (see Chapter 6).

138 PCR Protocols in Molecular Toxicology

Tailing Reaction

1. To 10 µl cDNA reaction add the following, on ice:

Component	µl	Final Concentration
ddH₂O	1	up to 20 µl
5 X Tailing buffer	4	1X
dATP (1 m*M*)	4	0.2 m*M*
Terminal d transferase	1	10 U

2. Incubate 5 min at 37°C and then 5 min at 65°C. Dilute to 200 µl with TE.

PCR Amplification

1. Prepare the PCR mix.

Note: *DMSO has been reported to aid in reducing secondary structure of DNA. This is particularly useful when trying to amplify regions with a high G:C content. This supplement may be removed and replaced with an additional 5 µl of ddH₂O.*

Component	µl	Final Concentration
ddH₂O	24–29	up to 50 µl
10 X PCR buffer	5	1X
DMSO	5	10%
dATP (100 m*M*)	0.75	1.5 m*M*
dCTP (100 m*M*)	0.75	1.5 m*M*
dGTP (100 m*M*)	0.75	1.5 m*M*
dTTP (100 m*M*)	0.75	1.5 m*M*
dT$_{17}$-Adapter primer (10 pmol/µl)	1µl	10 pmol
Adapter primer (10 pmol/µl)	3 µl	30 pmol
Gene-specific reverse primer (10 pmol/µl)	3 µl	30 pmol
cDNA pool	1–5	

Note: *The gene-specific reverse primer may be identical to that used in the cDNA reaction above. However, better specificity may be obtained if a sequence upstream is used for amplification.*

Cloning by PCR

2. Denature PCR mix at 85°C for 3 to 5 minutes. Add 2.5 units of *Taq* polymerase (0.5 µl/tube).

3. Place the reactions in the thermocycler only when it has reached at least 85°C. A sample PCR reaction is given below. The temperature, times, and cycles may need to be optimized for each primer pair.

Cycle (1X)

Denature	94°C 4 min
Anneal	55°C 5 min
Elongate	72°C 30 min

Cycle (30X)

Denature	94°C 20 sec
Anneal	55°C 30 sec
Elongate	72°C 2 min

Elongate	72°C 5 min
Store	4°C

Cloning of RACE products

1. Continue amplification of 5′ and 3′ RACE products until enough DNA is obtained to clone.

2. Proceed with basic TA cloning as described above.

VI. Library Screening by PCR

Obtaining a full-length cDNA clone for a gene of interest from a phage or plasmid library is often a tedious process. The standard library screening approach[2] involves infecting bacteria with the library, plating onto agar, lifting and lysing the resultant plaques or colonies onto nitrocellulose membranes. Subsequently the membranes are hybridized with a radioactive DNA probe; positive plaques or colonies are isolated and rescreened until a pure population is obtained. After the secondary or tertiary screening of a plasmid library, restriction enzyme digestion is used to select the largest insert followed by sequencing to verify its identity. With positive phage plaques, similar isolation and sequencing techniques are slightly more difficult. However, many com-

140   PCR Protocols in Molecular Toxicology

mercially available phage libraries contain recombination sequences and helper viruses which are used for the isolation of a plasmid from the phage containing the cDNA of interest. The time and the expertise required to obtain the full-length cDNA has lead to the design of PCR-based methods. In addition, the capacious use of radioactivity in library screening may result in contamination problems and adds considerable expense.

The following procedures assume you have the following: 1) Some information on the sequence of interest. This sequence information can be based on amino acid sequence, partial cDNA sequence (i.e., clones obtained from differential display PCR), or may represent a conserved domain. 2) A library that contains the cDNA of interest. Several commercial libraries are available from a variety of species and tissues. In addition, the construction of cDNA libraries has become easier with the advent of complete kits for cDNA synthesis, ligation into lambda phage arms, and packaging into virus.

Three similar methods of library screening by PCR are given below. Each involves multiple PCR amplifications and library dilutions. Protocol 3 is analogous to 5′ and 3′ RACE techniques discussed previously, but uses phage sequences in place of the anchored or adapter primers. These procedures can be used for either phage or plasmid libraries.

Protocol 1 — Dilution Screening

This procedure is based on reference 14.

1. Dilute the library to 10^5 plaque forming units (pfu)/5 μl or 10^5 colony forming units (cfu)/5 μl for phage or plasmid libraries, respectively, into ten tubes (labeled A through J). Water or SM buffer may be used as the diluent. A final volume of 1 mL is sufficient.

2. Prepare the following PCR mix in the order given.

Component	Final Concentration	1X	nX
ddH$_2$O	—	27	
MgCl$_2$ (25 mM)	3 mM	6	
10X PCR buffer	1X	5	
dATP (100 mM)	0.4 mM	0.2	
dCTP (100 mM)	0.4 mM	0.2	
dGTP (100 mM)	0.4 mM	0.2	
dTTP (100 mM)	0.4 mM	0.2	
Forward primer (10 pmol/μl)	0.6 nM	3	
Reverse primer (10 pmol/μl)	0.6 nM	3	

Cloning by PCR 141

Note: *The forward and reverse primer sequences may be gene specific (i.e., if partial cDNA sequence is known) or degenerate (i.e., if amino acid sequence is known or if a conserved domain is to be screened). However, if degenerate primers are used, more than 10 tubes may be required. See Section IV for considerations when designing degenerative primers.*

3. Place PCR mix at 85°C for at least 3 min. Meanwhile, pipet 5 µl of the diluted library into individual PCR tubes.

4. Add the equivalent of 0.25 µl *Taq* DNA polymerase (5 U/µl) per reaction to the preheated PCR mix. (For example, if 10 reactions are to be performed, add 2.5 µl *Taq*.)

5. Briefly heat PCR tubes containing bacterial lysate to 85°C in a heat block or thermocycler. Add 45 µl PCR mix with *Taq* to each DNA sample. Cap and vortex samples.

6. Immediately amplify using the following cycle profile (Perkin Elmer 9600 or equivalent):

Denature   94°C 4 min
            <u>Cycle (28X)</u>

Denature   94°C 20 sec
Anneal   59°C 30 sec
Elongate   72°C 30 sec

Elongate   72°C 5 min
Store   4°C

7. Add 5.5 µl 10X loading dye and resolve the PCR products on an agarose gel as described in Chapter 6. Identify which pools (A through J) produce the appropriately sized PCR product.

8. Dilute the pooled library(s) that contains the PCR product of interest 1:100 in ddH$_2$O. (i.e., 10 µl pooled cDNA plus 990 µL ddH$_2$O). Pipet 100 µl of this diluted library into a 96-well PCR plate(s). (Alternatively, a microtiter plate may be used.)

Note: *Label all diluted library samples carefully as they may be used subsequently for library screening with other primer sets.*

9. Twenty pooled aliquots will be prepared, representing the eight rows and twelve columns of the microtiter plate. Label twenty microfuge tubes with the pool label (A through J) plus R1 through R8 (rows) and C1 through C8 (columns). Remove 10 µl from each tube in a row and combine in the appropriate microfuge tube (80 µl final volume). Similarly, remove 10 µl for each tube in a column and place in the appropriate microfuge tube (120 µl total).

142 PCR Protocols in Molecular Toxicology

10. Amplify 5 µl of each of the subpooled libraries (i.e., AR1 through AC8) as described in Steps 2 through 7, but increase the number of PCR cycles to 30 to 32. Identify the single tube in the 96-well plate that produces the appropriate size PCR product. This will be the tube that is found in the positive column and positive row. This tube contains approximately 200 pfu or cfu/µl.

Note: *If a positive clone in this screen is not found, take an aliquot of the diluted subpool (i.e., 10 µl or 2000 pfu) and infect (if using a phage library) or transform (if using a plasmid library) a bacterial host. Plate onto agar, grow overnight, and elute into LB (plasmid) or SM (phage) buffer. Use 10 mL per plate. Aliquot the broth containing the enriched libraries directly into a 96-well plate at 100 µl to each well and repeat Steps 2 through 10.*

11. Dilute this positive tube 1:100 in ddH$_2$O and place 100 µl/well into a 96-well PCR tray. (Each tube now represents 2 pfu or cfu/µl). Repeat Steps 2 through 10. (Great care must be taken in labeling the 96-well trays and microfuge tubes. Dilutions should be named for the well from which they were derived.) Increase the number of cycles in the PCR reaction to 32 to 36.

12. Once a well in this second 96-well plate is discovered, the clone must be expanded to get enough to verify. Infect or transform the appropriate bacterial host using 10 µl from the positive well in this secondary 96-well plate. Plate onto an agar dish and grow overnight.

13. With a sterile toothpick or pipet tip pick 30 plaques or colonies. Proceed with PCR clone check as discussed in Section VIII.

Protocol 2 — Enrichment Screening by PCR

This procedure is based on reference 15.

1. Plate the cDNA library at 50,000 pfu or cfu/150 mm LB plate according to the supplier's instructions. Incubate plates at 37°C for 6 to 8 h or until plaques and colonies are clearly visible. At this concentration, 20 plates are required to obtain 1×10^6 plaques or colonies.

2. Add 10 mL SM buffer per plate and incubate at 4°C overnight or at 37°C for 2 h.

3. Collect the SM buffer in a 15 mL centrifuge tube. Centrifuge at $5000 \times g$ for 10 minutes. Remove supernatant to fresh tubes.

4. Add 40 µl chloroform to each tube and store at 4°C. A 5 µl aliquot of this stock will be used in the PCR reaction.

5. Prepare the following PCR mix in the order given.

Component	Final Concentration	1X	nX
ddH$_2$O	—	27	

Cloning by PCR

MgCl$_2$ (25 mM)	3 mM	6
10X PCR buffer	1X	5
dATP (100 mM)	0.4 mM	0.2
dCTP (100 mM)	0.4 mM	0.2
dGTP (100 mM)	0.4 mM	0.2
dTTP (100 mM)	0.4 mM	0.2
Forward primer (10 pmol/µl)	0.6 nM	3
Reverse primer (10 pmol/µl)	0.6 nM	3

Note: *The forward and reverse primer sequences may be gene specific (i.e., if partial cDNA sequence is known) or degenerate (i.e., if amino acid sequence is known or if a conserved domain is to be screened). However, if degenerate primers are used, more than 10 tubes may be required.*

6. Place PCR mix at 85°C for at least 3 min. Meanwhile, pipet 5 µl of the SM stock into individual PCR tubes.
7. Add the equivalent of 0.25 µl *Taq* DNA polymerase (5 U/µl) per reaction to the preheated PCR mix. (For example, if 20 reactions are to be performed, add 5 µl *Taq*.)
8. Briefly heat PCR tubes containing bacterial lysate to 85°C in a heat block or thermocycler. Add 45 µl PCR mix with *Taq* to each DNA sample. Cap and vortex samples.
9. Immediately amplify using the following cycle profile (Perkin Elmer 9600 or equivalent).

Denature	94°C 4 min
	Cycle (28X)
Denature	94°C 20 sec
Anneal	59°C 30 sec
Elongate	72°C 30 sec
Elongate	72°C 5 min
Store	4°C

10. Add 5.5 µl 10X loading dye and resolve the PCR products on an agarose gel as described in Chapter 6. Identify which library plate produced the appropriately sized PCR product.

144   PCR Protocols in Molecular Toxicology

11. For the secondary screen, replate the positive aliquot at approximately 300 pfu or cfu/100 mm plate. Repeat Steps 2 through 10 except use 4 mL of SM buffer and 15 µl of chloroform. It may be necessary to examine 10 to 20 plates to obtain a positive in the secondary screen.

12. The tertiary screen is performed from a positive secondary aliquot as described above.

13. Once a secondary aliquot is identified that contains a positive signal, replate this aliquot at approximately 300 pfu or cfu/100 mm LB agar dish. Grow for 6 to 8 h at 37°C.

14. With a sterile pipet tip pick several plaques from this plate and place in 100 µl SM buffer. Incubate at 4°C overnight or 37°C for 2 h.

15. Remove 5 µl from each of the phage stocks for PCR analysis as described in Steps 5 through 10.

16. The phage stock that contains the positive plaque may be expanded for plasmid or phage purification by reinfecting bacteria. Consult the supplier's technical manual for details on large-scale lysate production and plasmid excision.

Protocol 3 — Library RACE

1. Dilute the phage or plasmid library to approximately 10^6 pfu or cfu/µl.

2. Prepare the following PCR mix in the order given.

Component	Final Concentration	1X	nX
ddH$_2$O	—		27
MgCl$_2$ (25 mM)	3 mM		6
10X PCR buffer	1X		5
dATP (100 mM)	0.4 mM		0.2
dCTP (100 mM)	0.4 mM		0.2
dGTP (100 mM)	0.4 mM		0.2
dTTP (100 mM)	0.4 mM		0.2
Gene-specific primer (10 pmol/µl)	0.6 nM		3
Plasmid/phage-specific primer (10 pmol/µl)	0.6 nM		3

Note: *The gene-specific primers may be either forward or reverse primers. For 5' RACE, use a reverse gene-specific primer (reverse complement of coding strand) and a plasmid forward primer. For 3' RACE, a gene-specific forward primer and a plasmid reverse primer are used. Primers used for sequencing from plasmids (T7, SP6, M13(-20), M13(rev), etc.) make good choices for the plasmid-specific sequences. A nested primer design as discussed for conventional RACE may be required for the gene-specific primers.*

Cloning by PCR   **145**

3. Place PCR mix at 85°C for at least 3 min. Meanwhile, pipet 5 µl of the diluted phage into individual PCR tubes.

4. Add the equivalent of 0.25 µl *Taq* DNA polymerase (5 U/µl) per reaction to the preheated PCR mix. (For example, if 5 reactions are to be performed, add 1.25 µl *Taq*.)

5. Briefly heat PCR tubes containing the library to 85°C in a heat block or thermocycler. Add 45 µl PCR mix with *Taq* to each DNA sample. Cap and vortex samples.

6. Immediately amplify using the following cycle profile (Perkin Elmer 9600 or equivalent).

Denature   94°C 4 min
              <u>Cycle (28X)</u>

Denature   94°C 20 sec
Anneal   59°C 30 sec
Elongate   72°C 30 sec

Elongate   72°C 5 min
Store   4°C

7. Add 5.5 µl 10X loading dye and resolve the PCR products on an agarose gel as described in Chapter 6.

8. Remove unincorporated primers and nucleotides using any of the methods described in Chapter 6.

9. Dilute the purified PCR product 1:100 and reamplify as discussed above. If possible, nested gene-specific primers should be used to increase confidence in obtaining the proper product.

10. Purify the PCR product and proceed with TA cloning as discussed above.

VII. Examination of DNA-Protein Interactions. Selection and Binding Sites (SAAB) Technique

A. General Considerations

The study of protein–DNA interactions has been examined indirectly in the previous chapter through the examination of altered gene expression. In these types of studies it is implied that protein–DNA interactions are occurring, which is regulating the transcription of the target gene. In the present section,

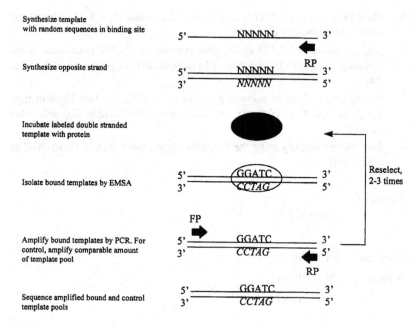

Figure 4.2
Selection and binding sites (SAAB) technique. A library of double-stranded oligonucleotides is prepared, and gel retardation assays are used to screen for DNA–protein interactions. After several rounds of selection, the sequence-specific oligonucleotides may be sequenced.

we will examine the direct interaction of protein with DNA through the use of a binding site library and electrophoretic mobility shift assays (EMSA). The interaction of the protein of interest with the DNA will be the criteria used to screen the library, and PCR will be used to enrich the selected oligonucleotides (see Figure 4.2). The exciting feature of the selection and binding sites (SAAB) technique[16] is the fact that RNA or DNA binding sites for any protein that binds selectively to a particular sequence can be examined. There need not be any indication of which genes this sequence is found in or if the protein–DNA interaction has a biological role. The SAAB technique is an ideal screening tool either for detecting a new interaction or assessing the role of mutations/alterations in a known binding site for the protein.

It is beyond the scope of this book to discuss how the protein of interest is isolated. We will assume that the DNA binding protein is cloned and can be either *in vitro* expressed or overproduced in baculovirus or bacteria. Rabbit reticulocyte lysate *in vitro* transcription and translation systems (i.e., Promega's TnT kit) provide a simple method to produce the protein of interest. For simplicity, we will also assume that the protein binds as monomer or homodimer. Of course, if the accessory proteins for a DNA-binding complex are known, they can be added to the incubations. The EMSA assays themselves are becoming commonplace in molecular toxicology labs. We will discuss a very basic assay system, which may require optimization for certain protein–DNA interactions.

Cloning by PCR

147

Protocol

DNA binding site library synthesis

1. Synthesize the following oligonucleotides:

   Oligo 1: 5' Oligo2-(N$_{13}$)-<u>Oligo3</u> 3'
   Oligo 2: 5' Clamp-Restriction site 1-(6-9 bases) 3'
   Oligo 3: 5' Clamp-Restriction site 2-(6-9 bases) 3'

Note: *N represents any of the four bases. <u>Oligo 3</u> is the reverse complement of Oligo 3. That is, Oligo 3 is the reverse primer, and Oligo 2 the forward primer of subsequent PCR reactions. A clamp is usually two to three bases of sequence that holds the double-stranded DNA together so that the restriction enzymes can cut more effectively (i.e., GC or ATA). The restriction endonucleases used should be good end-cutters and allow for easy cloning into an appropriate vector. The six to nine bases of sequence at the end of oligo 2 and oligo 3 can be taken directly from the 3' end of any primer pair that has been used effectively in your laboratory. Use a primer selection program to make sure that the two oligonucleotides are compatible with each other. Examples of Oligo 1, 2, and 3 are given in Blackwell and Weintraub[17] as well as Swanson et al.[18]*

2. The library of double-stranded binding sites is generated by the Klenow fragment of DNA polymerase. Assemble the following on ice. Incubate at 37°C for 1 h.

Component	µl	Final Concentration
Klenow 10X buffer	2.5	1X
dATP (10 mM)	0.5	0.2 mM
dCTP (10 mM)	0.5	0.2 mM
dGTP (10 mM)	0.5	0.2 mM
dTTP (10 mM)	0.5	0.2 mM
Oligo 1 (10 ng/µl)	2	20 ng
Oligo 3 (100 ng/µl)	10	100 ng
ddH$_2$O	16.5	
Klenow DNA polymerase	1	5 U

3. Purify the double-stranded probe by agarose gel electrophoresis excision and freeze-and-squeeze (Chapter 6).

PCR Protocols in Molecular Toxicology

4. Assemble the end-labeling reaction as follows:

Component	µl	Final Concentration
Double-stranded Oligo 1 (approx. 25 ng/µl)	2	50 ng
10X T4 polynucleotide kinase buffer	1	1X
[γ-^{32}P]ATP (3000 Ci/mmol at 10 mCi/ml)	1	—
ddH$_2$O	5	—
T4 polynucleotide kinase (10 U/µl)	1	10 U
Total volume	10	

5. Incubate at 37°C for 20 min. Stop the reaction by adding 1 µl 0.5 M EDTA.
6. Remove unincorporated nucleotide by G25 spin columns (i.e., ChromaSpin columns, Clontech). The final concentration of double-stranded, labeled Oligo 1 is approximately 5 ng/µl.

First Round Selection (Gel Shift Assay)

1. Assemble the following binding reactions in sterile microfuge tubes in the order shown:

ddH$_2$O	To a final volume of 10 µl
Gel shift 5X buffer	2 µl
DNA binding protein	Approximately 200 ng

2. Incubate the reactions at room temperature for 10 min.
3. Add 2 µl (10 ng and approximately 50,000 to 200,000 cpm) of ^{32}P-labeled Oligo 1 probe. Incubate the reactions at room temperature for 20 min.
4. Add 1 µl 10X loading dye and analyze the products as discussed below.

Electrophoresis of DNA-Protein Complexes

The reactions are resolved on nondenaturing, 4% acrylamide (30:1 acrylamide:bisacrylamide) gels. The format for the given example is for a 10×12 cm gel, 0.75 mm thick.

1. Assemble the following components in the order given. Cast and pour the gel according to the manufacturer's instructions. Allow at least two hours to polymerize.

Cloning by PCR

Component	Volume
ddH$_2$O	15.9 mL
10X TBE	1 mL
2% bisacrylamide	0.5 mL
40% acrylamide	2.0 mL
80% glycerol	625 µl
TEMED	10 µl
10% ammonium persulfate	150 µl

2. Prerun the gel in 0.5X TBE for 30 min at 100 V before loading the samples.

3. Load the samples. For the first round selection, run the gel until the bromophenol blue band has migrated approximately 1.5 cm. (For subsequent rounds of selection, the bromophenol blue band is allowed to migrate 8 cm.)

4. Wrap the gel in Saran® Wrap and expose to X-ray film. Upon developing the film, it should be apparent that the free probe has migrated with the dye front. In the first-round selection, a distinct "shifted" band, representing the protein-DNA complex, may not be readily visible.

Note: *The gel may be placed on Whatman 3MM paper and vacuum dried prior to exposing to X-ray film. In subsequent elution steps, the gel and the 3MM paper are cut and placed in elution buffer.*

5. Carefully cut a 1 cm segment from the gel, avoiding the free probe and remaining in the lane where the sample was loaded. This may be accomplished by using a razor blade and cutting through the X-ray film and the gel concurrently.

6. The slice is placed in 0.5 ml elution buffer (10 mM Tris-HCl (pH 8.0), 1 mM EDTA, 50 mM NaCl, and 0.2% SDS) and incubated for 3 h at 37°C. A small aliquot of the eluate may be used to determine the recovery of ^{32}P-labeled Oligo 1. Remove the eluate to a fresh tube.

7. Add 10 µg glycogen (used as a carrier), and 50 µl phenol:chloroform:isoamyl alcohol (25:24:1). Vortex and centrifuge for 10 minutes at 14,000 × g.

8. Remove the top phase to a fresh tube. Add 50 µl phenol:chloroform:isoamyl alcohol (25:24:1). Vortex and centrifuge for 10 minutes at 14,000 × g.

9. Remove the top phase to a fresh tube and add 250 µl ice cold 100% ethanol. Place at –20°C for 30 min. Centrifuge at 14,000 × g for 15 min. Remove the supernatant and gently dry the pellet. Resuspend in 25 µl ddH$_2$O. This sample constitutes the *Selected Library*.

Amplification of Selected DNA Pool

1. Prepare the following PCR mix in the order given.

150 PCR Protocols in Molecular Toxicology

Component	Final Concentration	1X
ddH$_2$O	—	20
MgCl$_2$ (25 mM)	3 mM	6
10X PCR buffer	1X	5
dATP (10 mM)	0.4 mM	2
dCTP (10 mM)	0.4 mM	2
dGTP (10 mM)	0.4 mM	2
dTTP (10 mM)	0.4 mM	2
Oligo 2 (10 pmol/µl)	0.6 nM	3
Oligo 3 (10 pmol/µl)	0.6 nM	3

2. Place PCR mix at 85°C for at least 3 min. Meanwhile, pipet 5 µl of the selected library to a PCR tube.

3. Add 0.5 µl *Taq* DNA polymerase (5 U/µl) to the preheated PCR mix.

4. Briefly heat PCR tubes containing the library to 85°C in a heat block or thermocycler. Add 45 µl PCR mix with *Taq* to each DNA sample. Cap and vortex samples.

5. Immediately amplify using the following cycle profile (Perkin Elmer 9600 or equivalent).

Denature	94°C 4 min
	<u>Cycle (26X)</u>
Denature	94°C 20 sec
Anneal	55°C 30 sec
Elongate	72°C 30 sec
Elongate	72°C 5 min
Store	4°C

6. Add 5.5 µl 10X loading dye and resolve the PCR products on an agarose gel. Gel purify the amplified band as described Chapter 6.

Subsequent Rounds of Selection

The PCR product from Step 6 above is used as the gel shift probe in the subsequent steps.

Cloning by PCR
151

1. Label the gel-purified, amplified Oligo 1 (Step 6 above) using a 1-cycle PCR as shown below:

Component	Final Concentration	1X
ddH$_2$O	—	6.7
MgCl$_2$ (25 mM)	3 mM	2.5
10X PCR buffer	1X	2
[γ-^{32}P]ATP (3000 Ci/mmol at 10 mCi/ml)	20 μCi	2
dCTP (10 mM)	0.4 mM	0.8
dGTP (10 mM)	0.4 mM	0.8
dTTP (10 mM)	0.4 mM	0.8
Oligo 2 (10 pmol/μl)	0.6 nM	1.2
Oligo 3 (10 pmol/μl)	0.6 nM	1.2

2. Add 0.5 μl *Taq* DNA polymerase (5 U/μl) to the PCR mix.
3. Pipet 2 μl amplified Oligo 1 (Step 6 above, diluted to 2.5 ng/μl) into the PCR mix which contains the *Taq*. Place immediately in the thermocycler and run the following program (Perkin Elmer 9600 or equivalent):

Denature	94°C 4 min
	<u>Cycle (1X)</u>
Denature	94°C 20 sec
Anneal	55°C 30 sec
Elongate	72°C 30 sec
Elongate	72°C 5 min
Store	4°C

4. Remove unincorporated nucleotide using G25 spin columns.
5. Proceed with the gel-shift assays, electrophoresis of DNA-protein complexes, and amplification of selected pools. The only adjustment made from the first round selection is the length of time of the electrophoresis (allow the dye to move 8 cm) and the fact that specific complexes are visualized and excised.
6. Typically three to four rounds of selection are required before discrete bands are seen in the gel-shift analysis.
7. The selected, amplified bands are subjected to digestion with restriction enzymes 1 and 2, following the supplier's instructions. (Sites for restriction enzymes 1

152   PCR Protocols in Molecular Toxicology

and 2 were included in Oligo 1, as well as Oligo 2 and Oligo 3.) The digested fragment may now be cloned and sequenced as discussed in Chapter 6.

VIII. PCR Clone Check

One of the essential techniques in molecular biology is to clone pieces of DNA into plasmid vectors. The ligation reaction, transformation of bacteria, and plating of cells onto agar plates has been discussed in several other portions of this book. A critical question is, how can you tell which bacterial colonies harbor the proper DNA fragment? A common method used to answer this question includes isolating small batches of plasmid, followed by restriction endonuclease digestion. This procedure requires growing the colonies in a liquid culture overnight, followed by often tedious plasmid purification. In the following procedure, the sensitivity of PCR is exploited to examine a very small number of bacteria. The bacterial colonies are stabbed with a toothpick or pipet tip and placed in water. Following lysis of the cells with heat, the plasmid is released into the water, where PCR is able to be used effectively to examine the identity of the insert (insert-specific primers) or the length of the insert (plasmid-specific primers).

Protocol

1. Perform the ligation and transformation reactions as usual. Grow the bacteria on agar plates with the appropriate antibiotic until colonies are distinct, with no satellite colonies.

Note: *Satellite colonies usually do not contain the plasmid, but grow close to a colony that does contain resistance. Avoid these smaller colonies surrounding a large, plasmid-containing central colony.*

2. Pipet 50 µl ddH$_2$O into the appropriate number of microfuge tubes. Generally, ten tubes per ligation reaction is sufficient. Prepare an agar plate with the appropriate antibiotic to serve as a master plate. Label the underside of the plate identically to the microfuge tubes.

3. With a sterile toothpick or pipet tip, perform the following in succession:

    i. Scrape a colony with the toothpick. Try to choose colonies that are well separated from surrounding colonies.

    ii. Stab the labeled agar plate (plus the appropriate antibiotic) with the toothpick

    iii. Place the toothpick in the microfuge tube containing 50 µl ddH$_2$O. Gently twirl the toothpick and discard.

4. Place the master plate inverted in a 37°C incubator, overnight.

Note: *After the overnight growth, the bacterial master plate may be stored in a refrigerator for up to two weeks. Once a positive colony is*

Cloning by PCR

153

observed, a sterile toothpick or pipet tip may be used to scrape the edge of the colony on the master plate for overnight growth.

5. Place the microfuge tubes in a 95°C heat block for 5 to 10 minutes. Place on ice for a moment and centrifuge briefly to remove condensate from the top of the tube.

6. Assemble the following in the order listed. (Either gene-specific primers or plasmid-specific primers may be utilized in this approach. With gene-specific primers, perform the optimized PCR protocol. The following procedure works well for most gene-specific primers as well as plasmid-specific primers, such as T7, SP6, and T3 sequencing primers).

Assemble the following in the order listed.

Component	Final Concentration	1X	nX
ddH$_2$O	—	27	
MgCl$_2$ (25 mM)	3 mM	6	
10X PCR buffer	1X	5	
dATP (100 mM)	0.4 mM	0.2	
dCTP (100 mM)	0.4 mM	0.2	
dGTP (100 mM)	0.4 mM	0.2	
dTTP (100 mM)	0.4 mM	0.2	
Forward primer (10 pmol/µl)	0.6 nM	3	
Reverse primer (10 pmol/µl)	0.6 nM	3	

7. Place PCR mix at 85°C for at least 3 min. Meanwhile, pipet 5 µl of the bacterial lysate into individual PCR tubes. Add one tube of 5 µl ddH$_2$O as a blank.

8. Add the equivalent of 0.25 µl *Taq* DNA polymerase (5 U/µl) per reaction to the preheated PCR mix. (For example, if 20 reactions are to be performed, add 5 µl *Taq*.)

9. Briefly heat PCR tubes containing bacterial lysate to 85°C in a heat block or thermocycler. Add 45 µl PCR mix with *Taq* to each DNA sample. Cap and vortex samples.

10. Immediately amplify using the following cycle profile (Perkin Elmer 9600 or equivalent):

Denature	94°C 4 min
	<u>Cycle (28X)</u>
Denature	94°C 20 sec

154   PCR Protocols in Molecular Toxicology

Anneal   59°C 30 sec
Elongate   72°C 30 sec

Elongate   72°C 5 min
Store   4°C

11.   Add 5.5 µl 10X loading dye and resolve the PCR products on an agarose gel
as described in Chapter 6. Identify colonies that produce the appropriately sized
PCR product.

Note: *The identity of the PCR product may be verified by digesting the PCR
product with an appropriate restriction endonuclease. Choose an
enzyme that will produce a minimal amount of easily resolved products. The PCR buffer is compatible with many restriction enzymes.
Add the 10X restriction enzyme buffer and enzyme directly to the PCR
reaction and incubate for 1 h at the optimal temperature.*

IX.   Direct Sequencing by PCR

DNA molecules or fragments (single-stranded, double-stranded, and plasmid
DNA) can be directly sequenced by combining PCR technology and the
dideoxynucleotide chain termination methods. This is a very powerful technique that is widely used in biotechnology, medicine, and other molecular
biological studies. There are also several sequencing kits available from commercial companies that are highly recommended for the beginner.

These methods assume that you have isolated a plasmid which contains
the sequence of interest. It is recommended that restriction enzyme mapping
be used to ensure that the appropriate insert is to be examined. Also, since the
polyacrylamide gels used in these procedures are very difficult to handle, it is
suggested that this particular step be practiced before radioactivity is used.

Protocol

This procedure is based on reference 19.

1.   Label four 0.5-ml microcentrifuge tubes (A, G, T, and C) for each set of
sequencing reactions for each primer. A, G, T, and C represent the terminators
ddATP, ddGTP, ddTTP, and ddCTP, respectively.
2.   Add 0.5 µl of 2X stock mixture of dNTPs/ddATP, dNTPs/ddGTP, dNTPs/ddTTP,
and dNTPs/ ddCTP to the labeled tubes A, G, T, and C, respectively. Add 0.5
µl ddH$_2$O to each tube, generating 1X working mixture solution. Cap the tubes
and store on ice until use.

Cloning by PCR

3. Prepare the following mixture for each set of four sequencing reactions for each primer in a microcentrifuge tube (0.5 ml) on ice.

   - Appropriate primer (15mer to 27mer, 10 to 30 ng/µl), 2 to 5 pmol (15 to 27 ng) depending on the size of primer
   - DNA template (0.4 to 7 Kb, 10 to 100 ng/µl), 100 to 1000 ng depending on the size of the template
   - $[\alpha\text{-}^{35}S]dATP$ (>1000 Ci/mmol), 1 to 1.2 µl
   - or $[(\alpha\text{-}^{32}P]dATP$ (800 Ci/mmol), 0.5 µl
   - 5X sequencing buffer, 4 µl
   - Add ddH$_2$O to a final volume of 17 µl

4. Add 1 µl (5 units/CL1) of sequencing-grade *Taq* DNA polymerase, i.e., (Promega Corporation) to the mixture at Step 3. Gently mix by pipetting up and down, and store on ice.

5. Remove 4 µl of the primer–template–enzyme mixture at Step 4 and add to the bottom of each tube containing 1 µl of dNTPs and the appropriate ddNTP prepared in Step 2.

6. Place the tubes in a thermal cycler preheated to 95°C and begin 30 cycles following the cycling profiles given in Table 4.3, depending on the size of primer and the size of DNA template.

7. After the PCR cycling is completed, add 3.5 µl of stop solution to inactivate the enzyme activity.

8. The reaction mixture can be directly subjected to electrophoresis following denaturation at 75°C for 2 min, or stored at 4°C until use. Load 3 µl per well. The procedures for electrophoresis and autoradiography are described elsewhere.

Reagents Needed

Any of the PCR buffers may be used in PCR. Buffer A may be used in both reverse transcriptase and PCR steps.

10X PCR Buffer A

   670 mM Tris-HCl, pH 8.8
   160 mM (NH$_4$)$_2$SO$_4$
   8 µM EDTA
   3% β-mercaptoethanol
   1 mg/ml bovine serum albumin (nuclease free)

10X PCR Buffer B

   500 mM KCl
   100 mM Tris-HCl, pH 9.0 (at 25°C)
   1.0% Triton X-100

TABLE 4.3
Thermal Cycling Profiles

Profile	Predenaturation	Cycling			Last
		Denaturation	Annealing	Extension	
Template (4 Kb); primer is <24 bases or with G-C content <40%	94°C, 2 min	94°C, 1 min	50°C, 1 min	70°C, 1.5 min	4°C
Template is >4 Kb; primer is >24mer or <24 bases with G-C content >50%	95°C, 2 min	95°C, 1 min	60°C, 1 min	72°C, 2 min	4°C

Cloning by PCR

10X PCR Buffer C
100 mM Tris-HCl, pH 8.3
500 mM KCl
0.1% BSA

5X MMLV Buffer
250 mM Tris-HCl, pH 8.3
375 mM KCl
15 mM MgCl$_2$

10X Transcription Buffer
800 mM HEPES-KOH, pH 7.5
240 mM MgCl$_2$
20 mM Spermidine
400 mM DTT

10X Ligase Buffer
300 mM Tris-HCl, pH 7.8
100 mM MgCl$_2$
100 mM DTT
10 mM ATP

10X Forward Exchange Buffer
0.5 M Tris-HCl, pH 7.5
0.1 M MgCl$_2$
50 mM DTT
1 mM Spermidine

10X T4 Polynucleotide Kinase Buffer
500 mM Tris-HCl, pH 7.5
100 mM MgCl$_2$
50 mM DTT
1 mM Spermidine
1 mM EDTA

TE Buffer
10 mM Tris-HCl, pH 8.0
1 mM EDTA

0.5 M EDTA

Chloroform/phenol (1:1)

Mix equal parts TE buffer and phenol and allow phases to separate. Then mix 1 part of the lower phenol phase with one part chloroform. Store in dark at 4°C.

PCR Primers

Dilute stock primers to 100 pmol/µl in ddH$_2$O and store at –70°C

For a working stock, dilute to 10 pmol/µl and store at –20°C

SM Buffer

50 mM Tris-HCl, pH 7.5
100 mM NaCl
8 mM MgSO$_4$
0.01% Gelatin
Sterilize by autoclaving

LB (Luria-Bertaini) Medium

Bacto-tryptone (10 g)
Bacto-yeast extract (5 g)
NaCl (5 g)
Adjust the pH to 7.5 with 2 N NaOH solution and autoclave. When it has cooled, store at 4°C until use. Make 4 liters

LB Plates

Add 15 g agar per liter unautoclaved LB medium. Adjust the pH to 7.5 with 2 N NaOH solution. Autoclave. When it has cooled to 50 to 55°C, add 50 µg/ml ampicillin, 0.5 mM IPTG, and 40 µg/ml X-Gal. Mix well and pour into LB plates (30 to 35 ml per plate) in a sterile laminar flow hood. Cover the plates and allow to harden for 1 h. Let the plates set at room temperature for 2 days before use. The plates can be placed at room temperature for up to 10 days, or wrapped and stored at 4°C for up to 1 month. The plates should be placed at room temperature prior to use.

Gel Shift 5X buffer

20% glycerol
5 mM MgCl$_2$
2.5 mM EDTA

Cloning by PCR

  2.5 mM DTT
  250 mM NaCl
  50 mM Tris-HCl, pH 7.5
  0.25 mg/ml poly(dI-dC)-poly(dI-dC)

6X Buffer (EMSA loading dye)

  0.25% bromophenol blue
  0.25% xylene cyanol FF
  30% glycerol in H_2O

2X dNTPs/ddATP Mixture

  dATP (80 μM)
  dTTP (80 μM)
  dCTP (80 μM)
  7-Deaza dGTP (80 μM)
  ddATP (1.4 mM)

2X dNTPs/ddTTP Mixture

  dATP (80 μM)
  dTTP (80 μM)
  dCTP (80 μM)
  7-Deaza dGTP (80 μM)
  ddTTP (2.4 mM)

2X dNTPs/ddGTP Mixture

  dATP (80 μM)
  dTTP (80 μM)
  dCTP (80 μM)
  7-Deaza dGTP (80 μM)
  ddGTP (120 μM)

2X dNTPs/ddCTP Mixture

  dATP (80 μM)
  dTTP (80 μM)
  dCTP (80 μM)
  7-Deaza dCTP (80 μM)
  ddCTP (800 μM)

5X Sequencing Buffer

  0.25 M Tris-HCl, pH 9.0 at room temperature
  10 mM MgCl$_2$

Stop Solution

10 mM NaOH
95% Formamide
0.05% Bromophenol blue
0.05% Xylene cyanol

10X Ficoll Loading Buffer

30% Ficoll in TE buffer
0.25% Bromophenol blue
0.25% Xylene cyanol (optional)

References

1. **Finney, M., Nisson, P.E., and Rachtchian, A.,** Molecular cloning of PCR products. *Current Protocols in Molecular Biology,* 15.7.1–15.7.11, 1995.
2. **Sambrook, J., Fritsch, E.F., and Maniatis, T.,** *Molecular Cloning, A Laboratory Manual,* 2nd ed., Cold Spring Harbor Press, Cold Spring Harbor, NY, 1989.
3. **Hengen, P.N.,** Cloning PCR products using T-vectors, *TIBS,* 20, 85, 1995.
4. **Kaufman, P.B., Wu, W., Kim, D., and Cseke, L.J.,** cDNA cloning by RT-PCR, in *Handbook of Molecular and Cellular Methods in Biology and Medicine,* Kaufman et al., Eds., CRC Press, Boca Raton, FL, 1995, 250.
5. **Scharf, S.J.,** Cloning with PCR, cloning with PCR, in *PCR Protocols: A Guide to Methods and Applications,* Innis et al., Eds., Academic Press, San Diego, 1990, 84.
6. **Jung, V., Pestka, S.B., and Pestka, S.,** Cloning of polymerase chain reaction-generated DNA containing terminal restriction endonuclease recognition sites, *Meth. Enzym.,* 218, 357, 1993.
7. **Compton, T.,** Degenerate primers for DNA amplification, in *PCR Protocols: A Guide to Methods and Applications,* Innis et al., Eds., Academic Press, San Diego, 1990, 30.
8. **Telenius, H., Carter, N.P., Bebb, C.E., Nordenskjöld, M., Ponder, B.A., and Tunnacliffe, A.,** Degenerate oligonucleotide-primed PCR: General amplification of target DNA by a single degenerate primer, *Genomics,* 13, 718, 1992.
9. **Peterson, M. and Tjian, R.,** Cross-species polymerase chain reaction: Cloning of TATA box-binding proteins, *Meth. Enzymol.,* 218, 493, 1993.
10. **Pytela, R., Suzuki, S., Breuss, J., Erle, D.J., and Sheppard, D.,** Polymerase chain reaction cloning with degenerate primers: Homology-based identification of adhesion molecules, *Meth. Enzymol.,* 245, 420, 1994.
11. **Sells, M.A. and Chernoff, J.,** Polymerase chain reaction cloning of related genes, *Meth. Enzymol.,* 254, 184, 1995.
12. **Martin-Parrar, L. and Zerial, M.,** Using oligonucleotides for cloning Rab proteins by polymerase chain reaction, *Meth. Enzymol.,* 257, 189, 1995.

Cloning by PCR

13. **Frohman, M.A.,** RACE: Rapid amplification of cDNA ends, in *PCR Protocols: A Guide to Methods and Applications,* Innis et al., Eds., Academic Press, San Diego, 1990, 28.

14. **Takumi, T. and Lodish, H.F.,** Rapid cDNA cloning by PCR screening, *BioTechniques,* 17, 443, 1994.

15. **Amaravadi, L. and King, M.W.,** A rapid and efficient, nonradioactive method for screening recombinant DNA libraries, *BioTechniques,* 16, 98, 1994.

16. **Blackwell, T.K.,** Selection of protein binding sites from random nucleic acid sequences, *Meth. Enzymol.,* 254, 604, 1995.

17. **Blackwell, T.K. and Weintraub, H.,** Differences and similarities in DNA-binding preferences of MyoD and E2A protein complexes revealed by binding site selection, *Science,* 250, 1104, 1990.

18. **Swanson, H.I., Chan, W.K., and Bradfield, C.A.,** DNA binding specificity and pairing rules of the Ah receptor, ARNT, and SIM proteins, *J. Biol. Chem.,* 26292, 1995.

19. **Kaufman, P.B., Wu, W., Kim, D., and Cseke, L.J.,** Direct sequencing by PCR, in *Handbook of Molecular and Cellular Methods in Biology and Medicine,* Kaufman et al., Eds., CRC Press, Boca Raton, FL, 1995, 233.

Chapter 5

Genotype Analysis

Douglas Bell and Gary Pittman

Contents

I. General Strategies and Applications.. 163
    A. Genotyping of Carcinogen Metabolism
       Polymorphisms 164
    B. High-Throughput Genotyping.. 165
II. Analysis of Polymorphisms Using PCR 167
    A. PCR-RFLP Genotyping for *NAT2* 167
       1. General Considerations 167
       2. PCR Protocol... 169
       3. Restriction Digest Protocol 170
       4. Results of RFLP Analysis 171
    B. Multiplex PCR Genotyping for *GSTM1* and *GSTT1* 172
       1. General Considerations 172
       2. PCR Protocol... 173
Materials Needed 174
References 175

I. General Strategies and Applications

The analysis of polymorphisms and mutations has classically been an area in
which PCR has flourished. In fact, many of the basic techniques discussed in
Chapter 1, and to some extent Chapter 4, have been developed in the context
of analyzing for these variations in the genome. In this section, we will discuss
basic approaches that may be used to examine base-pair changes in the DNA

0-8493-3344-X/98/$0.00+$.50
© 1998 by CRC Press LLC

163

164 PCR Protocols in Molecular Toxicology

sequence. The examples given may be adapted to the investigator's specific research interests.

A.   Genotyping of Carcinogen Metabolism Polymorphisms

Human genetic polymorphisms in metabolic activation and detoxification pathways appear to be important sources of inter-individual variation in susceptibility to cancer.[1] Individuals who inherit the "at-risk" alleles of genes for enzymes such as glutathione S-transferases (GST) and N-acetyltransferases (NAT) may fail to be protected against carcinogens in cigarette smoke, diet, industrial processes, and environmental pollution.[1-4]

This chapter briefly describes methods for detecting DNA sequence polymorphisms, which are *inherited* variations in a DNA sequence at a specific location in the genome (e.g., alternative nucleotides present at a specific position). These sequence variations can be base changes (referred to as single nucleotide polymorphisms, SNPs), deletions, duplications, or insertions, and these changes can occur in combinations. Sequence polymorphisms occur approximately every 800-bp in the human genome, so often they are within the coding region of a gene. Polymorphisms that alter protein function are of greatest interest, but detection of "silent" changes within the coding region or detection of noncoding intronic and flanking region polymorphisms can be useful in many applications (e.g., genetic linkage markers).

Polymorphisms often occur at restriction enzyme recognition sites and alter restriction enzyme digestion patterns, allowing detection by restriction fragment length polymorphism (RFLP) analysis. If PCR is carried out with primers that flank the polymorphic site, the PCR product contains the restriction site and can be digested with the diagnostic enzyme. The N-acetyltransferase 2 (*NAT2*) protocol in this chapter is an example of combining PCR with the RFLP technique (PCR-RFLP, Figure 5.1), a technique that has largely supplanted Southern blot-based RFLP genotyping. The mutant primer RFLP method is an approach that extends RFLP genotyping to sequence polymorphisms that contain only partial restriction sites. A mismatch is designed into the PCR primer in order to create a restriction site in the PCR product of one sequence variant but not the other (Figure 5.2). Digestion of the PCR product with the specific restriction enzyme allows deduction of the sequence at the restriction site. If possible, PCR primers for RFLP methods should flank a second nonpolymeric cutting site for the restriction enzyme. Cutting at this second position should always occur, and the presence of the constant band (Figure 5.2, 50-bp band in all lanes) serves as a positive control for the restriction digest.

If an SNP does not occur at a restriction site, allele-specific PCR (AS-PCR) is frequently used to detect the three possible genotypes. Two allele-specific primers are chosen, and a third common primer is designed to be used with either allele-specific primer (Figure 5.3). The AS-PCR primers are alike

Genotype Analysis

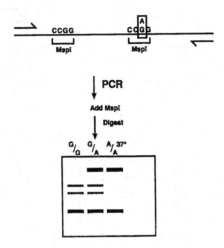

Figure 5.1
Polymerase chain reaction-restriction fragment length polymorphism (PCR–RFLP).

except that the 3' terminal nucleotide of one primer matches the wild-type allele (WT), and the 3' terminal nucleotide of the second primer matches the variant allele (MT). PCRs are carried out in parallel in separate tubes that include DNA from the test subject. Following PCR, the products are separated on agarose gels. Presence (or absence) of a band indicates the presence (or absence) of the wild-type or variant allele (Figure 5.3). Coamplification of a second, nonpolymorphic gene (e.g., β-globin) in the same PCR is often carried out as a positive control (see reference 2).

An unusual case of allele-specific PCR is used to detect the presence or absence of alleles containing deletions of genes in the GST gene family. Because the *GSTM1* and *GSTT1* genes have null alleles, in which the entire gene sequence is absent, one can use PCR primers that specifically amplify the functional allele. This allele-specific amplification indicates the presence of the gene and therefore, the GST genotype (Figure 5.4, method explained in Section II.B).[3,4]

B. High-Throughput Genotyping

Population-based studies are moving rapidly toward high-throughput genotyping methods, which potentially allow the processing of thousands of samples per day. Automation of sample handling steps and use of non-gel-based detection are making these approaches a reality. Technical developments in the area of genotyping are progressing rapidly, and microscale approaches involving high density deposition of oligonucleotide probes on silica chips are likely to be practical soon. However, relatively high throughput can be achieved with

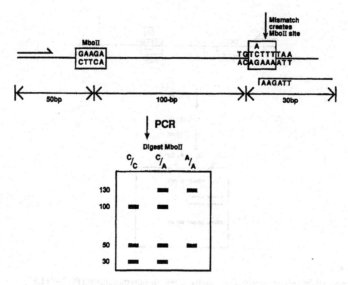

Figure 5.2
Mutant primer PCR.

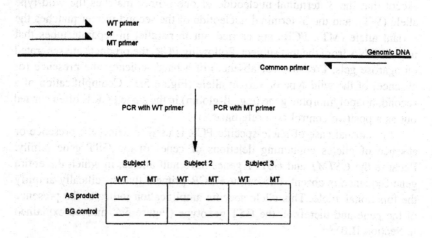

Figure 5.3
Allele-specific PCR.

existing gel-based methods. The use of multiplex PCR, which incorporates multiple primer sets into the same PCR reaction, can increase throughput by several fold. Most PCR machines allow the 96-well format and when this approach is combined with high resolution agarose in a long format, multi-comb, small well (5 µL) gel electrophoresis apparatus, large numbers of samples can be processed quickly. Systems allowing electrophoresis of more than 200 samples per gel are available.

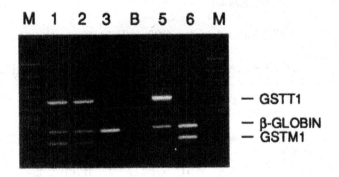

Figure 5.4
Agarose gel showing PCR fragments from multiplex PCR of *GSTM1*, *GSTT1*, β-globin genes. Lanes 1 and 2 show results from samples that are *GSTM1* and *GSTT1* positive; lane 3 shows a sample that is null for both *GSTM1* and *GSTT1*; lane 5 is null for *GSTM1*; lane 6 is null for *GSTT1*. The PCR fragment from the β-globin gene is present in all lanes (except the reagent blank lane, B; marker, M).

The PCR oligo-ligation assay (OLA) is an existing high-throughput, ELISA-based genotyping method that detects ligated allele-specific oligonucleotides.[5,6] Because the process is carried out entirely in 96-well microtiter plate format and detection is accomplished with a standard microplate reader, this method can easily be automated using robotic pipeting stations. While a thorough description of this method is beyond the scope of this chapter, investigators with plans to carry out more than 5000 genotypes per year may want to consider this approach.

The methods presented in this chapter are relatively simple gel-based genotyping approaches that can be used in small laboratories and require only basic equipment. The protocols for PCR-based polymorphism assays for *N*-acetyltransferase 2 (*NAT2*), glutathione S-transferase M1 *(GSTM1)*, and T1 *(GSTT1)* are presented as examples of genotyping. Understanding the concepts presented here should allow investigators to design methods that serve their own research needs.

II. Analysis of Polymorphisms Using PCR

A. PCR-RFLP Genotyping for *NAT2*

1. General Considerations

Figure 5.5 shows a diagram of the *NAT2* gene with the location of *NAT2* forward (-113 NAT2F) and reverse (996 NAT2R) PCR primers, locations of the various polymorphic nucleotides, and a map of the restriction enzyme sites. The primer sequences are:

NAT2 Forward primer (100pmol/μL) 5' cca ttg tgt ttt tac gta tt

NAT2 Reverse primer (100pmol/μL) 5' gta ttt gat gtt tag gat ttt

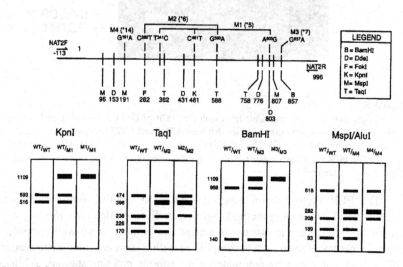

Figure 5.5
NAT2 genotyping using PCR–RFLP. Upper part of figure shows restriction enzyme map and position of polymorphic nucleotides that create the different slow acetylator alleles.

TABLE 5.1
NAT2 Restriction Site Changes and Allele Names

Allele	Change (nucleotide position)	Trivial name
NAT2*4	None	Wild-type, Rapid
NAT2*5	*Kpn* I site deleted (C481T)	M1
NAT2*6	*Taq* I site deleted (G590A)	M2
NAT2*7	*BamH* I site deleted (G857A)	M3
NAT2*14	*Msp* I site deleted (G191A)	M4

PCR primer locations for *NAT2* were chosen to allow for: 1) specific amplification of *NAT2* and not *NAT1* or *NATP* (*NAT* pseudogene), and 2) resolution of the digested PCR fragments on a 3% high-resolution agarose gel. Table 5.1

Genotype Analysis

indicates the restriction site changes that can be used to distinguish specific alleles. NAT gene nomenclature is complex, and further details can be obtained in references 7 and 8. PCR primers flank the gene and amplify a 1109-bp fragment. PCR is carried out as described below, is divided into four aliquots, and restriction enzymes are added. Combining digests in the same tube has been successful in some protocols and can increase throughput.[8] Electrophoretic separation of PCR products by electrophoresis on agarose gels results in patterns similar to those shown in the lower part of Figure 5.5.

2. PCR Protocol

1. Prepare a PCR tray with one sample tube for each DNA sample.
2. Pipet 10 μL of 0.01 μg/μL DNA (100 ng) into each sample tube, and cap the sample tubes.
3. Prepare the PCR mix by calculating the total reaction amount needed for each of the following reagents. Combine all components except the Taq DNA polymerase, and vortex the PCR mix tube.

Reagent	Amount per sample	Final Concentration
Sterile deionized H_2O	29.6 μL	
10X PCR buffer	5.5 μL	1X
$MgCl_2$ (25 mM)	4.4 μL	2.0 mM
dATP (10 mM)	1.1 μL	0.2 mM
dCTP (10 mM)	1.1 μL	0.2 mM
dGTP (10 mM)	1.1 μL	0.2 mM
dTTP (10 mM)	1.1 μL	0.2 mM
$NAT2$ forward primer (100 pmol/μL)	0.4 μL	0.73 pmol/μL
$NAT2$ reverse primer (100 pmol/μL)	0.4 μL	0.73 pmol/μL
Taq DNA polymerase (5 U/μL)	0.3 μL	0.027 U/μL

4. Incubate the PCR mix and the sample tray in a heat block at 85°C for at least 5 min.
5. Add the appropriate amount of Taq DNA polymerase to the PCR mix tube, vortex the tube, and place the tube back in the heat block.

170 PCR Protocols in Molecular Toxicology

6. Remove the caps from the sample tubes, and rapidly pipet 45 µL of the 85°C PCR mix into each sample tube.

7. Recap the sample tubes, and vortex the sample tray.

8. Quickly transfer the sample tray from the heat block to the idling 85°C thermocycler without letting the samples cool below 85°C.

9. Amplify using the following cycling profile:

| Initial denaturation | 94°C 4 min |
| | (26 to 30 cycles) |

Amplification

Denaturation	94°C 30 sec
Annealing	50°C 30 sec
Elongation	72°C 1 min 30 sec
Final elongation	72°C 4 min

10. After the PCR, 5 µL of each reaction may be run out on a 1 to 2% agarose gel to check if PCR amplification was successful.

Notes: *Although this protocol was designed as a hot start PCR performed on a Perkin-Elmer GeneAmp® PCR System 9600 thermocycler (or equivalent machine), it has been used successfully in a cold start format. The 55 µL total reaction volume provides four 10 µL digests and an additional 15 µL for PCR product testing and/or one additional (or repeat) digest. The reaction may be scaled up to larger volumes to provide additional RFLP digests. Also, when first attempting this protocol, one should perform the PCR with a range of MgCl$_2$ concentrations to ensure optimal PCR amplification. When using the 85°C hot start method, it is strongly recommended that one prepare an excess volume of the PCR mix (Section II.A.2, Step 3), typically enough for three to four extra reactions. Pipetting liquids at 85°C can lead to volume errors which, while not critical in terms of the success of the PCR, may result in insufficient PCR mix volume to complete the entire tray. Because PCRs rarely fail on a large scale, i.e., an entire tray of samples, one may choose to omit the testing of PCR product prior to digestion (Section II.A.2, Step 10) to save time and labor.*

3. Restriction Digest Protocol

1. Label one digest tray for each restriction digest, (i.e., 4 trays, *Kpn* I, *Taq* I, *BamH* I, and *Msp* I/*Alu* I). Each digest tray will have the same number of tubes as the number of PCR samples.

2. Aliquot 10 µL of each PCR sample into each digest tray.

Genotype Analysis

3. Prepare the restriction digest mix by calculating the total reaction amount needed for each of the following reagents. For each digest mix, combine all components except the enzymes, vortex the digest mix tube, and place the tube on ice.

Kpn I *Digest Mix*	*Amount per sample*	*Taq* I *Digest Mix*	*Amount per sample*
10X *Kpn* I buffer	1.5 µL	10X *Taq* I buffer	1.5 µL
Sterile deionized H_2O	2.5 µL	Sterile deionized H_2O	2.5 µL
Kpn I (10 U/µL)	1 µL	*Taq* I (10 U/µL)	1 µL

BamH I *Digest Mix*	*Amount per sample*	*Msp* I/*Alu* I *Digest Mix*	*Amount per sample*
10X *BamH* I buffer	1.5 µL	10X *Msp* I/*Alu* I buffer	1.5 µL
Sterile deionized H_2O	1.5 µL	Sterile deionized H_2O	1.5 µL
BamH I (10 U/µL)	2 µL	*Msp* I (10 U/µL)	1 µL
		Alu I (10 U/µL)	1 µL

4. Add *Kpn* I, *Taq* I, *BamH* I, and *Msp* I/*Alu* I to the respective digest mixes, vortex each tube, and place on ice.

5. Aliquot the appropriate *per sample* amount of the digest mix to each respective digest tray tube, cap tubes, and vortex the digest trays.

6. Incubate the *Taq* I digest tray at 65°C for 1 to 2 h.

7. Incubate the *Kpn* I, *BamH* I, and *Msp* I/*Alu* I digest trays at 37°C for 4 to 16 h.

8. Prepare a 3% agarose gel with 10 µL ethidium bromide (10 mg/mL).

9. Add 5 µL of loading dye to each digested sample.

10. Load 10 to 15 µL of each digested sample on the gel.

11. Run the *Kpn* I, *Taq* I, *BamH* I, and *Msp* I/*Alu* I digest products at 80 to 120 volts for 1 to 3 h.

Notes: The amounts of restriction enzymes listed in Section II.A.3 represent an excess of enzyme (5 to 10 units/sample) relative to the amount of PCR product typically produced. One may wish to use lesser amounts of enzymes; however, it is recommended that a range of at least 1 to 5 units/sample be used. When analyzing the NAT2 RFLP PCR digestion product on an agarose gel, one should avoid using agarose concentrations of more than 3% because the BamH I digest may be difficult to resolve at higher concentrations.

4. Results of RFLP Analysis

The restriction digests are specific for the *NAT2* alleles shown in Table 5.1.

The possible restriction patterns for genotypes are shown in Figure 5.5. For each DNA sample tested, one first determines the genotype for each restriction digest (as shown in Table 5.2). By comparing results for all digests, one can determine the composite genotype and phenotype. Subject 1 has one nonfunctional allele (M1), is heterozygous, and therefore has an intermediate rapid genotype. Subject 2 has both M2 and M3 alleles and has a slow phenotype, while for subject 3 the results show only the presence of functional (wt) alleles at each polymorphic site.

TABLE 5.2
Interpretation of NAT2 Restriction Digest Results (Examples)

	Kpn I	Taq I	BamH I	Msp I	Genotype	Phenotype
Subject 1	wt/M1	wt/wt	wt/wt	wt/wt	wt/M1	Intermediate Rapid
Subject 2	wt/wt	wt/M2	wt/M3	wt/wt	M2/M3	Slow
Subject 3	wt/wt	wt/wt	wt/wt	wt/wt	wt/wt	Rapid

B. Multiplex PCR Genotyping for GSTM1 and GSTT1

1. General Considerations

As mentioned earlier, the phenotypic absence of glutathione S-transferase Mu 1 (*GSTM1*) and Theta 1 (*GSTT1*) enzyme activity in humans is due to the presence of a homozygous, inherited deletion of the gene termed the null genotype. One detects the presence of these genes by amplifying highly specific regions of these two genes using multiplex PCR, which is the use of multiple sets of primers in a single PCR (Figure 5.4). The primer sequences are:

*GST M*1 Forward primer (100pmol/µL) 5′ gaa ctc cct gaa aag cta aag c

*GST M*1 Reverse primer (100pmol/µL) 5′ gtt ggg ctc aaa tat acg gtg g

*GST T*1 Forward primer (100pmol/µL) 5′ ttc ctt act ggt cct cac atc tc

*GST T*1 Reverse primer (100pmol/µL) 5′ tca ccg gat cat ggc cag ca

BG Forward primer (100pmol/µL) 5′ caa ctt cat cca cgt tca cc

BG Reverse primer (100pmol/µL) 5′ gaa gag cca agg aca ggt ac

Genotype Analysis **173**

The presence of a band on the agarose gel indicates the presence of one or two copies of the gene in the genomic DNA sample. The absence of a band indicates an individual homozygous for the null allele. In addition to *GSTM*1 and *GSTT*1 primers, a set of primers for the β-globin gene are added to the multiplex PCR as a positive control for amplification.

2.   PCR Protocol

1.   Prepare a PCR tray with one sample tube for each DNA sample.
2.   Pipet 5 μL of 0.01 μg/μL DNA (50 ng) into each sample tube, and cap the sample tubes.
4.   Prepare the PCR reaction mix by calculating the total reaction amount needed for each of the following reagents. Combine all components except the *Taq* DNA polymerase, and vortex the PCR mix tube.

Reagent	*Amount per sample*	*Final Concentration*
Sterile deionized H_2O	4.72 μL	
10X PCR buffer	1.5 μL	1X
$MgCl_2$ (25 m*M*)	2 μL	3.3 m*M*
dATP (10 m*M*)	0.3 μL	0.2 m*M*
dCTP (10 m*M*)	0.3 μL	0.2 m*M*
dGTP (10 m*M*)	0.3 μL	0.2 m*M*
dTTP (10 m*M*)	0.3 μL	0.2 m*M*
*GSTM*1 Forward primer (100 pmol/μL)	0.1 μL	0.67 pmol/μL
*GSTM*1 Reverse primer (100 pmol/μL)	0.1 μL	0.67 pmol/μL
*GSTT*1 Forward primer (100 pmol/μL)	0.1 μL	0.67 pmol/μL
*GSTT*1 Reverse primer (100 pmol/μL)	0.1 μL	0.67 pmol/μL
BG Forward primer (100 pmol/μL)	0.05 μL	0.33 pmol/μL
BG Reverse primer (100 pmol/μL)	0.05 μL	0.33 pmol/μL
Taq DNA polymerase (5 U/μL)	0.08 μL	0.020 U/μL

4.   Incubate the PCR mix and the sample tray in a heat block at 85°C for at least 5 minutes.
5.   Add the appropriate amount of *Taq* DNA polymerase to the PCR mix tube, vortex the tube, and place the tube back in the heat block.

PCR Protocols in Molecular Toxicology

6. Remove the caps from the sample tubes, and rapidly pipet 10 μL of the 85°C PCR mix into each sample tube.

7. Recap the sample tubes, and vortex the sample tray.

8. Quickly transfer the sample tray from the heat block to the idling 85°C thermocycler without letting the samples cool below 85°C.

9. Amplify using the following cycling profile:

Initial denaturation	94°C 4 min
	(26–30 cycles)
Amplification	
Denaturation	94°C 10 sec
Annealing	62°C 30 sec
Elongation	72°C 45 sec
Final elongation	72°C 4 min

10. Prepare a 3% agarose gel with 10 μL ethidium bromide (10 mg/mL).

11. After PCR, add 5 μL of loading dye to each sample tube and load on gel.

Notes: *Although this protocol was designed as a hot start PCR performed on a Perkin-Elmer GeneAmp PCR System 9600 thermocycler (or equivalent machine), it has been successfully used in a cold start format. We have also used a commercially available Taq DNA polymerase antibody (TaqStart™ Antibody, Clontech Laboratories, Inc.) for complete PCR setup at room temperature. When first attempting this protocol, one should perform the PCR with a range of $MgCl_2$ concentrations to ensure optimal PCR amplification. When using the hot start method, it is strongly recommended one prepare an excess volume of the PCR mix (Section II.B.2, Step 3), typically enough for three to four extra reactions. Pipetting liquids at 85°C can lead to volume errors which, while not critical in terms of the success of the PCR, may result in insufficient PCR mix volume to complete the entire tray.*

Materials Needed

For both PCR assays described, the following materials are needed:

- 96-well PCR reaction tray (e.g., Perkin-Elmer MicroAmp® Reaction Tray/Retainer)
- 0.2 mL PCR reaction tubes and caps (e.g., Perkin-Elmer MicroAmp® Reaction Tubes)
- Sterile deionized H_2O

Genotype Analysis

- 10X PCR buffer

  For ten 1 mL aliquots, combine the following:
  219.4 mg ammonium sulfate
  6.7 mL 1 M Tris (pH 8.8 in DEPC-treated H_2O)
  1 mL EDTA (25 mg/100 mL in DEPC-treated H_2O)
  35 μL β-mercaptoethanol
  8 mg BSA
  H_2O up to 10 mL
  Mix well and divide into 1 mL aliquots.
  Store at −20°C.

- $MgCl_2$ (25 mM)
- dATP (10 mM)
- dCTP (10 mM)
- dGTP (10 mM)
- dTTP (10 mM)
- *Taq* DNA polymerase (5 U/μL)
- Agarose (e.g., FMC NuSieve® 3:1)
- Ethidium bromide (10 mg/mL)
- Loading dye
  Add 50 μL 1% xylene cyanol to 1 mL 30% Ficoll in H_2O.

Additionally for the *NAT2* RFLP assay, the following materials are needed:

- *Kpn* I (10 U/μL) and compatible buffer
- *Taq* I (10 U/μL) and compatible buffer
- *BamH* I (10 U/μL) and compatible buffer
- *Msp* I (10 U/μL) and compatible buffer
- *Alu* I (10 U/μL) and compatible buffer

References

1. **Bell, D.A., Taylor, J.A., Butler, M.A., Stephens, E., Wiest, J., Brubaker, L., Kadlubar, F., and Lucier, G.W.,** Genotype/phenotype discordance for human arylamine N-acetyltransferase (NAT2) reveals a new slow-acetylator allele common in African-Americans, *Carcinogenesis,* 14, 1689, 1993.
2. **Bell, D.A., Stephens, E., Castranio, T., Umbach, D.M., Watson, M., Deakin, M., Elder, J., Duncan, H., Hendrickse, C., and Strange, R.C.,** Polyadenylation polymorphism in the *N*-acetyl-transferase gene 1 (*NAT1*) increases risk of colorectal cancer, *Cancer Research,* 55, 3537, 1995.

PCR Protocols in Molecular Toxicology

3. Bell, D.A., Taylor, J.A., Paulson, D., Robertson, D., Mohler, J., and Lucier, G.W., Genetic risk and carcinogen exposure: A common inherited defect of the carcinogen metabolism gene glutathione transferase M1(GSTM1) is associated with increased susceptibility to bladder cancer, *J. Nat. Cancer Inst.*, 85, 1159, 1993.

4. Chen, H., Sandler, D., Taylor, J.A., Shore, D.L., Liu, E., Bloomfield, C., and Bell, D.A., Increased risk for myelodysplastic syndromes among those with glutathione s-transferase theta 1 (GSTT1) gene defect, *Lancet*, 347, 295, 1996.

5. Innis, M.A., Gelfand, D., Sninsky, J., and White, T., *PCR Protocols*, Academic Press, San Diego, 1990.

6. Delahunty, C., Ankener, W., Deng, Q., Eng, J., and Nickerson, D., Testing the feasibility of DNA typing for human identification by PCR and an oligonucleotide ligation assay, *Am. J. Hum. Gen.*, 58, 1239, 1996.

7. Doll, M., Fretland, A., Deitz, A., and Hein, D., Determination of human NAT2 acetylator genotype by restriction fragment length polymorphism and allele specific amplification, *Anal. Biochem.*, 231, 413, 1995.

8. Vatsis, K., Weber, W., Bell, D.A., Dupret, J.-M., Evans, D.A.P., Grant, D., Hein, D., Lin, H., Meyer, U., Relling, M., Sim, E., Suzuki, T., and Yamazoe, Y., Nomenclature for N-acetyltransferases, *Pharmacogenetics*, 5, 1, 1995.

Chapter 6

General Molecular Biology Techniques

John P. Vanden Heuvel

Contents

I. Introduction 178
II. Isolation and Purification of Genomic DNA from Animals 179
 Protocol A — Extraction of Genomic DNA with Organic
 Solvents 179
 Protocol B — Genomic DNA Extraction by Formamide 181
 Reagents Needed 181
III. Isolation and Purification of Plasmid DNA 182
 A. Isolation of Plasmid DNA by Alkaline Lysis 183
 Protocol A — Mini-Preparation of Plasmid DNA 183
 Protocol B — Large-Scale Preparation of Plasmid DNA 184
 Reagents Needed 185
IV. Isolation and Purification of RNA 186
 A. Rapid Isolation of Total RNA 186
  1. Acid Guanidinium Thiocyanate-Phenol-Chloroform
   Method 186
  2. LiCl-Urea and Phenol-Chloroform Method 188
  3. Isolation of Total RNA with Guanidinium Thiocyanate
   and a CsCl Gradient 189
 B. Purification of Poly(A)+RNA from Total RNA 190
  1. Purification of mRNA by Oligo(dT)-Cellulose
   Column 190
  2. Mini-Purification of mRNA by Oligo(dT)-Cellulose
   Column 191

0-8493-3344-X/98/$0.00+$.50
© 1998 by CRC Press LLC

177

Reagents Needed	192

| C. | Measurement of RNA | 195 |

Protocol 195

V. Subcloning the DNA Fragment of Interest 196

A. Restriction Enzyme Digestion of Vector and DNA Insert for Subcloning 196

Protocol A — Preparation of Vectors..................................... 197

Protocol B — Preparation of Insert DNA............................... 198

Reagents Needed.. 198

B. Ligation of Plasmid Vector and Insert DNA 199

Protocol 199

C. Bacterial Transformation 200

Protocol A — Preparation of Competent Cells for CaCl$_2$ Transformation 201

Protocol B — Preparation of Competent Cells for Heat Shock Transformation 201

D. Transformation Using Heat Shock Method 201

Protocol 201

E. Transformation Using the CaCl$_2$ Method 202

F. Selection of Transformants Containing Recombinant Plasmids 202

Protocol 202

Reagents Needed.. 203

VI. Chloroform:Phenol Extraction of DNA 204

VII. Agarose Gel Electrophoresis of DNA 205

A. General Considerations 205

Protocol 206

B. Purifying DNA Fragments from Agarose Gels 207

1. Freeze-and-Squeeze Method 207

2. Elution from Wells of Agarose Gels............................... 208

Reagents Needed.. 208

VIII. Transfection of Mammalian Cells 209

Reagents Needed.. 211

References 211

I. Introduction

In this chapter we have tried to assemble a few methods that are needed in a variety of PCR-based procedures. These are basic methods common in molecular biology laboratories, and mastering these techniques is absolutely required for developing a successful PCR project. The reader is referred to Kaufman et al.[1] and Sambrook et al.[2] for more details.

General Molecular Biology Techniques   **179**

II. Isolation and Purification of Genomic DNA from Animals

This discussion is based on reference 1.

The following protocols describe the purification of animal DNA that is suitable for various procedures including PCR amplification and restriction enzyme digestion. In order to obtain high-molecular-weight DNA, certain precautions must be taken. To avoid DNase contamination, all glassware, plastic pipette tips, centrifuge tubes, cell scrapers, solutions, and buffers should be autoclaved or sterile-filtered. Molecular biology grade or ultrapure chemicals or reagents are strongly recommended. Vigorous shaking should be avoided to prevent DNA from shearing. Gloves should be worn during isolation procedures.

Protocol A — Extraction of Genomic DNA with Organic Solvents

1. Harvest tissue or collect cells and add lysis buffer to the samples.

    Extraction from fresh blood cells

    i.   Collect cells from fresh blood (20 ml per extraction) by centrifuging at 1000 rpm for 15 min at room temperature and carefully decant the supernatant (contains lysed red cells without nuclei)

    ii. Add 1 volume of phosphate-buffered saline (PBS) to the remainder (contains white blood cells) and centrifuge at 1000 rpm for 15 min at room temperature

    iii. Carefully decant the supernatant and resuspend the cells in 15 ml of acid citrate dextrose solution (ACD). Incubate at 37°C for 1 to 1.5 h prior to Step 2.

    Extraction from frozen blood cells

    i.   Thaw frozen blood sample (20 ml per extraction) in a water bath at 22°C and transfer the sample to a fresh centrifuge tube

    ii. Add an equal volume of PBS and centrifuge at 1200 rpm for 15 min at room temperature

    iii. Decant the supernatant (contains lysed red cells) and resuspend the white blood cells in 15 ml of ACD solution. Incubate the sample at 37°C for 1 to 1.5 h. Proceed to Step 2.

    Extraction from cells grown in monolayers

    i.   Rinse the confluent monolayers of cells twice with ice-cold PBS. Add 10 to 15 ml ice-cold PBS and carefully scrape the cells, using a sterile policeman or cell scraper, into a clean tube. Collect the cells by centrifugation at 1000 rpm for 10 min at 4°C.

    ii. Resuspend the cells in 8 volumes of ice-cold PBS and centrifuge at 1000 rpm for 10 min at 4°C. Resuspend the cells at 4×10^7 cells/ml in TE buffer.

180 PCR Protocols in Molecular Toxicology

    iii. Transfer the cell suspension to a clean tube or a flask and add 9 ml of lysis buffer per milliliter of the cell suspension. Incubate the mixture at 37°C for 1 to 1.5 h. Carry out Step 2.

Extraction from cells grown in suspension

    i. Collect the cells by centrifugation at 1000 rpm for 10 min at 4°C and wash them twice with 1 volume of ice-cold PBS without calcium. Recollect the cells by centrifugation at 1000 rpm for 10 min at 4°C.

    ii. Resuspend the cells at a concentration of 4×10^7 cells/ml in TE buffer (pH 8.0).

    iii. Add 10 volumes of lysis buffer and incubate at 37°C for 1 to 1.5 h. Proceed to Step 2.

Extraction from tissue

    i. Harvest fresh and soft tissue using sterile scissors or razor blade and immediately freeze in liquid nitrogen. Store at –80°C until use.

    ii. Grind the tissue in a clean mortar with pestle using liquid nitrogen. Keep adding liquid nitrogen and grinding until a fine powder is obtained. Allow the liquid nitrogen to evaporate for a few minutes, but never warm or thaw the powder too long before adding lysis buffer.

    iii. Transfer the powder, little by little, to a 30-ml Corex centrifuge tube or a sterile beaker containing 8 to 10 volumes of lysis buffer. Let the powder spread over the surface of the lysis buffer and gently shake to submerge the material. Incubate the tube at 37°C for 1 to 1.5 h. Proceed to Step 2.

2. Add proteinase K (20 mg/ml in ddH$_2$O) to a final concentration of 100 µg/ml of the lysed-cell suspension from Step 1 and gently mix well.

3. Incubate the mixture in a water bath at 50°C for 2 to 4 h. Gently swirl the viscous mixture every 20 min.

4. Allow the mixture to cool to room temperature and transfer the mixture into a Corex centrifuge tube. Add 1 volume of 0.5 M Tris-buffer (pH 8.0)-saturated phenol and mix well by gently inverting the tube for 5 min.

5. Centrifuge at $6000 \times g$ at room temperature for 15 min and carefully transfer the top, viscous, aqueous phase to a fresh tube with a wide-bore pipette.

6. Repeat phenol extraction (Steps 4 and 5) two more times.

7. Add 0.5 volume of 7.5 M ammonium acetate (pH 5.2) to the aqueous phase. Slowly pour the supernatant into a fresh tube or beaker containing 2 to 2.5 volumes (of the supernatant volume) of chilled 100% ethanol. Do not vortex or invert the tube or beaker until the DNA precipitate floats up to the surface of the ethanol (15 to 30 min at room temperature).

8. Centrifuge the DNA at $5000 \times g$ for 5 min at 4°C. Briefly and gently rinse the DNA with 4 ml of 70% ethanol and dry the sample under vacuum for 15 to 30 min.

9. Resuspend the DNA in an appropriate amount of TE buffer (1 ml/4×10^7 cells). If the DNA does not go into solution after 15 min at room temperature, the sample can be placed at 45 to 50°C for 15 to 30 min with gentle and occasional shaking until it is dissolved. Keep the tube open to let remaining ethanol evaporate. At this stage, the DNA should be very pure with a size of 100 to 200 Kb.

General Molecular Biology Techniques

10. Measure the quantity and quality of the DNA using a UV-visible spectrophotometer at the wavelengths of 260 and 280 nm (A_{260} and A_{280})

Note: *A pure DNA should have an A_{260}/A_{280} ratio of 1.85 to 2.0. A ratio of A_{260}/A_{280} less than 1.75 means that a significant amount of protein remains in the DNA sample. In this case, add SDS to a concentration of 0.5% to denature remaining proteins and extract the proteins by repeating Steps 2 through 10. Store the DNA sample at –20°C. The quality and size of the DNA preparation may be also checked by 0.3 to 0.8% of agarose gel electrophoresis, by pulsed-field gel electrophoresis, or by electrophoresis through a 0.3% agarose gel poured on a 1% agarose support.*

The concentration of a DNA sample is calculated as follows:

$$DNA\ (\mu g/\mu l) = A_{260} \times 50\ \mu g/ml \times dilution\ factor$$

Protocol B — Genomic DNA Extraction by Formamide

This is a relatively simple and low-cost method compared with Protocol A. The DNA isolated by this method has a molecular weight higher than 200 Kb, which is suitable for doing restriction enzyme digestion and PCR amplification. The procedures are described as follows:

1. Conduct Steps 1 through 3 as described in Protocol A.

2. Allow the suspension of lysed cells to cool to 15°C, and add 0.7 volume of denaturation buffer to the suspension. Gently mix using a glass rod, and place the mixture overnight at 15°C.

3. Pool and dialyze the viscous suspension in a collodion bag (Sartorius SM 13200E or equivalent) three times against 4 liters of buffer A and five times against 4 liters of buffer B.

4. Measure the quantity and quality of the DNA with a spectrophotometer at 260 and 280 nm (see Protocol A). A pure DNA should have an A_{260}/A_{280} ratio of 1.85 to 2.0. The sample can be stored at –20°C until used. If the ratio A_{260}/A_{280} is less than 1.75, repeat Steps 2 through 4.

5. The quality and size of the DNA preparation may be checked by 0.3 to 0.8% of agarose gel electrophoresis, by pulsed-field gel electrophoresis, or by electrophoresis through a 0.3% agarose gel poured on a 1% agarose support.

Reagents Needed

Lysis Buffer

> 10 mM Tris-HC1, pH 8.0
> 100 mM EDTA, pH 8.0

20 µg/ml Pancreatic RNase
0.5% SDS

PBS (pH 7.4) without Calcium

NaCl (8.07 g)
KCl (0.201 g)
Na_2HPO_4 (1.15 g)
KH_2PO_4 (0.204 g)
Dissolve well after each addition in 800 ml ddH$_2$O, adjust the
pH to 7.4, and add ddH$_2$O to a final volume of 1000 ml.
Autoclave.

ACD Solution

Citric acid (4.8 g)
Sodium citrate (13.2 g)
Glucose (14.7 g)
Adjust to a final volume of 1000 ml with ddH$_2$O.

Denaturation Buffer

80% Deionized formamide (v/v)
0.8 M NaCl
20 mM Tris-HC1, pH 8.0

Buffer A

0. 1 M NaCl
20 mM Tris-HCl, pH 8.0
10 mM EDTA, pH 8.0

Buffer B

10 mM NaCl
10 mM Tris-HC1, pH 8.0
1 mM EDTA, pH 8.0

III.   Isolation and Purification of Plasmid DNA

This section is based on reference 1.

Extraction and purification of plasmid DNA is an essential technique in
modern molecular toxicology studies. The isolation of large quantities of
plasmid is required for DNA sequencing (Chapter 4), TA cloning (Chapters
2, 3, and 4), subcloning (Chapter 4), and many other procedures not covered
in this book. Plasmids are usually purified from liquid cultures by inoculating

General Molecular Biology Techniques **183**

an appropriate volume of LB (Luria-Bertaini) medium with a single bacterial colony picked up from an agar plate. There are many methods currently applied to isolate plasmid DNA. We describe in detail two protocols that are very commonly used and successful in our and other laboratories. There are also many commercially available kits that can help the beginner get started. The reader is referred to reference 2 for a description of the appropriate microbiology techniques (i.e., plating bacteria, preparing LB plates, etc.).

A. Isolation of Plasmid DNA by Alkaline Lysis

This protocol allows for the rapid purification of small to large amounts of plasmid DNA without the need for cesium gradients, and is the most common method for plasmid purification. The principle of the procedure is: denature plasmid and chromosomal DNA under alkaline conditions and selectively renature plasmid DNA following neutralization of the solution. The isolated DNA is suitable for restriction enzyme digestion, *in vitro* transcription, DNA subcloning, and DNA sequencing. Although it is possible to avoid the chloroform:phenol extraction steps, the removal of bacterial proteins will increase the efficiency of subsequent reactions.

Protocol A — Mini-Preparation of Plasmid DNA

1. Inoculate a single colony or 10 µl of previously frozen cells containing the plasmid of interest in 5 ml LB medium with the appropriate antibiotics (e.g., ampicillin 50 µg/µl, see reference 2 for the concentration of other antibiotics) depending on the antibiotic-resistant gene carried by the specific plasmid. Culture the bacteria at 37°C overnight, shaking at 200 to 220 rpm.

2. Add 1.5 ml of the overnight culture to two microcentrifuge tubes and centrifuge at $10,000 \times g$ for 2 min. Remove the liquid and invert the tubes on a paper towel to dry the bacterial pellet for 4 min.

3. Resuspend the pellet by adding 0.1 ml of ice-cold lysis buffer and vortex for 2 min. Incubate the tubes for 5 min at room temperature.

4. Add 0.2 ml of a freshly prepared alkaline solution and mix by inversion 5 to 6 times. **Never vortex.** Incubate the tubes on ice for 5 min.

5. Add 0.15 ml of ice-cold potassium acetate solution. Mix by inversion for 20 sec and incubate on ice for 5 min. The purpose of this step is to selectively renature the plasmid DNA. Some chromosomal DNA may be partially renatured and bound by proteins, which will be extracted by phenol/chloroform in later steps.

6. Centrifuge at $12,000 \times g$ for 5 min and gently transfer the supernatant to fresh tubes.

7. Add RNase A (DNase-free) into the supernatant to a final concentration of 20 µg/ml. Incubate the tubes at 37°C for 20 min. RNase A degrades total RNA from the sample.

184 PCR Protocols in Molecular Toxicology

8. Add an equal volume of TE-saturated phenol/chloroform to each tube and mix by vortexing for 1 min.

9. Centrifuge at 12,000 × g for 4 min and transfer the upper, aqueous phase into fresh tubes.

10. Add an equal volume of chloroform:isoamyl alcohol (49:1) and mix by vortexing for 1 min and centrifuge as in Step 9.

11. Centrifuge at 12,000 × g for 4 min and transfer the supernatant to a fresh tube. Steps 8 through 11 act to remove RNase A, proteins, and DNA-protein complexes.

12. Add 2.5 volumes of 100% ethanol. Mix by inversion and allow the plasmid DNA to precipitate for 20 min at –80°C or 2 h at –20°C.

13. Centrifuge at 12,000 × g for 10 min. Decant the supernatant and briefly and gently rinse the pellet with 1 ml of pre-chilled 70% ethanol. Dry the plasmid DNA under vacuum for 20 min.

14. Dissolve the dried plasmid DNA in 25 µl of TE buffer or sterile deionized water. Take 2 to 4 µl to measure the concentration and store the sample at –20°C until use.

Protocol B — Large-Scale Preparation of Plasmid DNA

The principle is the same as the mini-preparation method but will yield up to 100 µg plasmid per 100 ml LB media. Of course, the yield will depend on the plasmid and, to some extent, the insert.

1. Inoculate a single colony or 50 µl of previously frozen cells containing the plasmid of interest in 100 ml of LB medium with the appropriate antibiotic (e.g., ampicillin 50 µg/µl, see reference 2 for the concentration of other antibiotics) depending on the antibiotic-resistant gene carried by the specific plasmid. Culture the bacteria at 37°C overnight, shaking at 200 to 220 rpm.

2. Add 30 ml of the overnight culture to two 30-ml Corex tubes and centrifuge at 9000 × g for 5 min at 4°C. Remove the liquid and invert the tubes on a paper towel to dry the bacterial pellet for 5 min. In the following steps, it is recommended that the two samples in two tubes always be processed separately.

3. Resuspend the pellet by adding 2 ml of ice-cold lysis buffer and vortex for 2 min. Incubate the tubes for 5 min at room temperature.

4. Add 4 ml of a freshly prepared alkaline solution and mix by inversion 5 to 6 times. **Do not vortex**. Incubate the tubes on ice for 5 min.

5. Add 3 ml of ice-cold potassium acetate solution, mix by inversion for 20 sec, and incubate on ice for 5 min.

6. Centrifuge at 10,000 × g for 5 min at 4°C and gently transfer the supernatant to fresh tubes.

7. Add RNase A (DNase-free) to the supernatant to a final concentration of 20 µg/ml. Incubate the tubes at 37°C for 30 min.

8. Add 1 volume of TE-saturated phenol/chloroform to each tube and mix by vortexing for 1 min.

General Molecular Biology Techniques

185

9. Centrifuge at 10,000 × g for 5 min at 4°C. Transfer the upper, aqueous phase into fresh tubes.

10. Add 1 volume of chloroform:isoamyl alcohol (49:1) and mix by vortexing for 1 min and centrifuge as in Step 9.

11. Centrifuge at 10,000 × g for 5 min at 4°C and transfer the supernatant to a fresh tube.

12. Add 2.5 volumes of 100% ethanol. Mix by inversion and allow the plasmid DNA to precipitate for 30 min at –80°C or 2 h at –20°C.

13. Centrifuge at 12,000 × g for 15 min at 4°C. Remove the supernatant, and gently rinse the pellet with 6 ml of pre-chilled 70% ethanol. Dry the plasmid DNA under vacuum for 20 min.

14. Dissolve the dried plasmid DNA in 200 µl of TE buffer or sterile deionized water. Take 25 µl to measure the concentration and store the sample at –20°C until use.

Reagents Needed

LB (Luria-Bertaini) Medium (per liter)

> 10 g Bacto-tryptone
> 5 g Bacto-yeast extract
> 5g NaCl
> Adjust pH to 7.5 with 2 N NaOH and autoclave. Add antibiotics after the autoclaved solution has cooled to less than 50°C.

TE Buffer

> 10 mM Tris-HCl, pH 8.0
> 1 mM EDTA

Lysis Buffer

> 25 mM Tris-HCl, pH 8.0
> 10 mM EDTA
> 50 mM Glucose

Denaturing Solution

> 0.2 N NaOH
> 1% SDS

Potassium Acetate Solution (pH 4.8)

> Prepare 120 ml of 5 M potassium acetate. Add 23 ml of glacial acetic acid and 57 ml of H_2O. Total volume is 200 ml. This solution is 3 M with respect to potassium and 5 M with respect to acetate. Store on ice until use.

DNase-Free RNase A

Make a 10-mg/ml solution of RNase A in 10 mM Tris-HCl, pH 7.5, and 15 mM NaCl. Heat at 100°C for 10 min and cool slowly to room temperature.

TE-Saturated Phenol/Chloroform

Thaw crystals of phenol in 65°C water bath with occasional shaking. Mix equal parts of TE buffer and thawed phenol. Let the mixture stand until the phases separate at room temperature. Mix an equal part of the lower, phenol phase with an equal part of chloroform:isoamyl alcohol (49:1).

IV. Isolation and Purification of RNA

The extraction of RNA is much more complicated than that of DNA because RNA is much more labile and the risk of RNase contamination is very high. Great care should be taken to avoid contamination with RNase. Fortunately, RT–PCR is a very forgiving technique and slightly degraded RNA may not be as catastrophic as in techniques such as Northern blots.

The two most common sources of RNase contamination are users' hands and airborne bacteria and fungi. Since this enzyme is very difficult to inactivate, care should be taken to prevent RNase contamination. Some precautions are given below.[1]

1. Gloves should be worn at all times and changed frequently.
2. Whenever possible, disposable plasticware should be autoclaved and used for RNA isolation. It is highly recommended to use disposable plasticware whenever possible.
3. Nondisposable glassware and plasticware should be treated with 0.1% diethyl pyrocarbonate (DEPC) in ddH$_2$O and be autoclaved prior to use. After treatment, glassware should be baked at 250°C overnight.
4. Inactivators of endogenous RNase such as 4 M guanidine thiocyanate and β-mercaptoethanol are strongly recommended for inclusion in the extraction buffer. Whenever possible, solutions should be treated with 0.05% DEPC at 37°C for 2 h or overnight at room temperature and then autoclaved for 30 min to remove any trace of DEPC. Tris buffers, which cannot be treated with DEPC, should be made in DEPC-treated ddH$_2$O.

A. Rapid Isolation of Total RNA

1. Acid Guanidinium Thiocyanate-Phenol-Chloroform Method

This protocol is based on reference 3.

General Molecular Biology Techniques

1. Homogenize the sample as suggested below.

For tissue

Harvest tissue and immediately drop in liquid nitrogen. Store at −70°C until use. Grind 1 g tissue with a mortar and pestle using liquid nitrogen. Keep adding liquid nitrogen and grinding until a fine powder is obtained. Transfer the powder with a sterile spatula into a clean 14- or 50-ml polypropylene tube. Add 10 ml of solution B, mix, and keep the tube on ice. Proceed to Step 2.

Alternatively, homogenize the tissue in 10 ml of solution B in a sterile polypropylene tube on ice by using a glass-Teflon® homogenizer or equivalent polytron at top speed for two 30-sec bursts. Transfer the homogenate to a fresh polypropylene tube and proceed to Step 2.

For cultured cells grown in suspension culture or in a monolayer

Collect 1 to 2×10^8 cells in a sterile 50-ml polypropylene tube by centrifugation at $400 \times g$ for 5 min at 4°C. Wash the cell pellet with 25 ml of ice-cold, sterile 1X PBS and centrifuge at $400 \times g$ for 5 min at 4°C. Repeat washing and centrifugation once more to remove all traces of serum. Serum contains RNase and can ruin the experiment, therefore, take great care in the washing steps. Remove the supernatant and resuspend in 10 ml solution B. Keep the tube on ice and homogenize the cell suspension using a microtip on a Polytron® for two 0.5- to 1-min bursts at top speed and carefully transfer homogenate to a fresh tube. Proceed to Step 2.

Caution: Guanidinium thiocyanate is a potent chaotropic agent and irritant.

2. Add the following to the sample in the order given:
   - 1 ml of 2 *M* sodium acetate buffer (pH 4.0)
   - 10 ml of water-saturated phenol
   - 2 ml of chloroform:isoamyl alcohol
   - Cap the tube and mix by inversion after each addition. Vigorously shake the tube for 20 sec

*Caution: Phenol is poisonous and can cause severe burns. Proper laboratory clothing including gloves and goggles should be worn when handling these reagents. If phenol contacts your skin, wash the area immediately with large volumes of water, but **do not rinse with ethanol!**[1]*

3. Centrifuge at 12,000 × g for 20 min at 4°C using a Corex tube or at 7000 to 8000 rpm for 30 to 40 min at 4°C using a 14-ml polypropylene tube in the swing-out rotor. Carefully transfer the top, aqueous phase to a fresh tube. Decant the phenol phase into a special container for disposal.

4. Add 10 ml of isopropanol, mix, and allow to precipitate at −20°C for 1.5 to 2 h.

PCR Protocols in Molecular Toxicology

5. Centrifuge at 12,000 × *g* for 20 min at 4°C using a Corex tube or at 7000 to 8000 rpm for 30 to 40 min at 4°C using a 14-ml polypropylene tube in the swing-out rotor. Resuspend the RNA pellet in 3 ml of solution B and add 3 ml of isopropanol. Mix and then place at –20°C for 2 h or overnight.

6. Centrifuge at 12,000 × *g* for 20 min at 4°C using a Corex tube or at 7000 to 8000 rpm for 30 to 40 min at 4°C using a 14-ml polypropylene tube in the swing-out rotor. Briefly rinse the total RNA pellet with 4 ml of 75% ethanol. Dry the pellet under vacuum for 15 min.

7. Dissolve the total RNA in 200 µl of 0.5% SDS solution or DEPC-treated water. Take 20 µl to measure the concentration with the spectrophotometer at 260 and 280 nm.

Note: *The ratio of A_{260}/A_{280} should be 1.8 to 2.0 to be considered a good RNA preparation. The RNA isolated may be checked by 1% agarose, formaldehyde denaturing gel electrophoresis. Two strong rRNA bands should be visible.*

8. The RNA sample may be stored at –80°C until use for poly(A)+RNA purification or for dilution to a working solution for RT–PCR.

2. LiCl-Urea and Phenol-Chloroform Method

This procedure is based on reference 1.

1. Homogenize tissue as shown below

For tissue

Harvest tissue and immediately drop in liquid nitrogen. Store at –70°C until use. Grind 1 g tissue in a clean blender or with a mortar and pestle using liquid nitrogen. Keep adding liquid nitrogen and grinding until a fine powder is obtained. Warm the powder at room temperature for a few minutes and immediately transfer the powder with a sterile spatula into a clean 14- or 50-ml polypropylene tube. Add 8 ml of RNA extraction solution, mix, and keep the tube on ice. Proceed to Step 2.

Alternatively, homogenize the tissue in 8 ml of RNA extraction solution in a sterile polypropylene tube on ice by using a glass-Teflon homogenizer or equivalent Polytron at top speed for two 30-sec bursts. Transfer the homogenate to a fresh polypropylene tube and proceed to Step 2.

For cultured cells grown in suspension culture or in a monolayer

Collect 1 to 2×10^8 cells in a sterile 50-ml polypropylene tube by centrifugation at 400 × *g* for 5 min at 4°C. Wash the cell pellet with 25 ml of ice-cold, sterile 1X PBS and centrifuge at 400 × *g* for 5 min at 4°C. Repeat washing and centrifugation once more to remove all traces of serum. Remove the supernatant and resuspend in 8 ml RNA extraction solution. Keep the tube on ice and

General Molecular Biology Techniques

homogenize the cell suspension using a microtip and a polytron for two 0.5-to 1-min bursts at top speed and carefully transfer the homogenate to a fresh tube. Proceed to Step 2.

2. Place the homogenate at 0 to 4°C for at least 4 h and then centrifuge at 3000 × g for 25 min at 4°C.

3. Remove the supernatant and add 0.5 volume of cold RNA extraction solution. Mix well by vortexing and centrifuge as in Step 2.

4. Carefully decant the supernatant and dissolve the pellet in RNA buffer.

5. Extract proteins, carbohydrates, DNA, and cellular debris with 1 volume of phenol:chloroform:isoamyl alcohol (25:24: 1). Shake for 5 min.

Caution: Phenol is toxic; gloves should be worn at all times.

6. Centrifuge at 10,000 × g for 10 min at 4°C and carefully remove the top, aqueous phase to a fresh tube. Avoid the interface between two phases (the white material) as this contains high concentration of proteins and some DNA. Repeat Steps 5 and 6 one more time.

7. Add 0. 1 volume of 3 M sodium acetate and 2 volumes of 100% chilled ethanol. Mix well and allow the RNA to precipitate at –20°C for 2 h or on dry ice for 20 min.

8. Centrifuge at 12,000 × g for 10 min at 4°C. Discard the supernatant and wash the RNA pellet with 4 ml of 70% ethanol. Dry the pellet under vacuum for 15 min and dissolve the total RNA in 50 μl of RNA buffer containing 0.2% SDS. Take 5 μl of the sample to measure the concentration of the RNA. Store the sample at –20°C until use for poly(A)+RNA purification. The RNA sample may be stored at –80°C until use for poly(A)+RNA purification or for dilution to a working solution for RT–PCR

3. Isolation of Total RNA with Guanidinium Thiocyanate and a CsCl Gradient

This procedure is based on reference 1.

1. Collect and transfer tissue or cells into a homogenizing tube. Add 5 volumes of 4 M guanidinium thiocyanate buffer to 1 g of tissue or to 2 × 10^7 cells/ml of cell suspension or confluent monolayer of cells.

2. Homogenize the tissue on ice with a Polytron homogenizer (RNase-free) or equivalent at top speed for two 1-min bursts.

3. Transfer the homogenate to a fresh tube and add sodium lauryl sarcosinate to a final concentration of 0.5% and mix well.

4. Centrifuge at 5000 × g for 10 min at room temperature. Carefully transfer the supernatant to a fresh tube.

5. Carefully layer the supernatant onto a cushion of CsCl/EDTA solution in a clear ultracentrifuge tube. Mark the position of the cushion on the outside of the tube. Add 4 M guanidinium thiocyanate homogenization buffer to fill the tubes and to equalize their weights.

PCR Protocols in Molecular Toxicology

TABLE 6.1
Swinging-Bucket Rotors Centrifugation

| | Speeds and Time | | |
| | Rotor types | | |
	SW60 (7/16" × 23")	SW40 (9/16" × 32")	SW28 (1/2" × 31")
Volume of CsCl/EDTA (ml)	1.2	3.5	12.0
Volume of homogenate (ml)	3.1	9.7	26.5
Time (h)	12	24	26
Speed (rpm)	40,000	32,000	23,500

6. Centrifuge at 20°C at the speed and for the time given in Table 6.1 using a swinging-bucket rotor.

7. Turn off the centrifuge brake before decelerating the rotor to prevent the contents of the tube from becoming disturbed. Carefully remove the tubes from the centrifuge. Using a Pasteur pipette, gently remove the fluid, little by little, above the level of the cushion containing the white, viscous cellular DNA. With a fresh pipette and an automatic pipettor, keep removing the gradient fluid until close to the bottom of the tube. Briefly invert the tube to drain away any remaining fluid with pieces of Kimwipe paper and return the tube to an upright position afterwards.

8. Briefly wash CsCl from the RNA pellet with 2 ml of 70% ethanol and dry the RNA pellet at room temperature. Dissolve the RNA in the 100 μl of water. Wash the ultracentrifuge tube with another 100 μl water and pool the RNA solutions together.

9. Transfer the RNA sample to a fresh tube with 0.1 volume of 3 M sodium acetate buffer and 2.5 volumes of chilled 100% ethanol. Mix well and allow the RNA to precipitate at –20°C for 2 h or more.

10. Centrifuge at 12,000 × g for 10 min at 4°C. Discard the supernatant. Briefly rinse the pellet with 70% ethanol. Dry under vacuum for 15 or 30 min by air in a laminar flow hood.

11. Dissolve the RNA in 50 μl of TE buffer. Take 5 μl of the sample to measure the concentration and quality of the RNA. Store the sample at –80°C until use.

B. Purification of Poly(A)+RNA from Total RNA

This procedure is based on reference 1.

1. Purification of mRNA by Oligo(dT)-Cellulose Column

1. Add 4 ml of binding buffer to 0.5 g of oligo(dT)-cellulose in a clean tube and mix well. Transfer the suspension to a 10-ml poly-prep chromatography column

General Molecular Biology Techniques

(Bio-Rad) or equivalent. Vertically fix the column in a holder with a clamp and place the column at 4°C for 2 h to equilibrate the cellulose resin.

2. Remove the column to room temperature and wash it by adding 2 ml of 0. 1 N NaOH solution through the top of the resin. The color of the resin changes from white to yellow. Allow the washing fluid to drain away by gravity and repeat washing the column five times.

3. Neutralize the column by adding 4 ml of binding buffer to the top of the resin and drain away the binding buffer by gravity. The color of the resin returns to white. Repeat five times and store at 4°C until use.

4. Add 1 volume of loading buffer to the total RNA sample prepared. Heat the mixture for 10 min at 65°C to denature the secondary structure of RNA, and then allow the sample to cool to room temperature.

5. Slowly load the total RNA sample to the top of the column capped at the bottom and allow the sample to run through the column by gravity. Gently loosen the resin in the column and let the column stand for 5 min. Remove the bottom cap to drain away the fluid from the bottom of the column and collect the fluid containing some unbound mRNA. Reload the fluid onto the column to allow the unbound mRNA to bind to the oligo(dT)-cellulose column and collect the eluate. Repeat this one more time.

6. Wash the column with 2 ml of washing buffer each time and drain away the buffer. Repeat washing three times.

7. Cap the bottom of the column and add 1 ml of elution buffer to the column to elute bound poly(A)+RNA. Gently loosen the resin using a clean needle and allow the column to stand for 4 min. Remove the bottom cap and collect the eluate in a clean tube. Elute the column twice with 1 ml of elution buffer and collect the eluate.

8. Pool the eluates together and add 0. 15 volume of 3 M sodium acetate and 2.5 volumes of 100% chilled ethanol to precipitate the mRNA. Mix and place at –20°C overnight.

9. Centrifuge at $12,000 \times g$ for 15 min at 4°C. Decant the supernatant and briefly wash the mRNA pellet with 2 ml of 70% ethanol. Dry the pellet under vacuum for 15 min to remove ethanol and dissolve the mRNA in 20 to 50 µl of TE buffer. Take 2 or 4 µl of the sample to measure the concentration of the mRNA. At this stage, the sample should have a ratio of A_{260}/A_{280} of 1.9 to 2.0. The quality of the purified mRNA may be checked by 1% agarose, formaldehyde-denaturing gel electrophoresis. A broad-range smear should be visible from the top to the bottom of the well with or without two weak rRNA bands. The yield of poly(A)+RNA may be expected to be approximately 6% of total RNA. Store the sample at –70°C until use.

2. Mini-Purification of mRNA by Oligo(dT)-Cellulose Column

1. Add 1 ml of binding buffer to 0.3 g of oligo(dT)-cellulose in a microfuge tube. Mix and place at 4°C for 30 min.

192   PCR Protocols in Molecular Toxicology

2. Wash the resin with 1 ml of 0.1 N NaOH solution and mix gently for a few minutes. Centrifuge at $1500 \times g$ for 2 min and discard the supernatant and repeat this step eight times.

3. Neutralize the resin with 1 ml of binding buffer and gently mix with a sterile needle. Centrifuge at $1500 \times g$ for 2 min and carefully decant the supernatant. Repeat this step eight times. Resuspend the resin with 1 ml of binding buffer.

4. Add 1 volume of loading buffer to 100 μl of the total RNA sample (about 2 μg/μl). Heat the mixture for 10 min to 65°C and allow to cool to room temperature.

5. Load the total RNA sample to the 1 ml slurry of oligo(dT)-cellulose prepared in Step 3. Gently shake for 2 min and place at room temperature for 15 min to allow the RNA to bind to the resin.

6. Centrifuge at $1500 \times g$ for 5 min and carefully remove the supernatant.

7. Add 0.5 ml of wash buffer to the resin and gently shake for 10 sec. Centrifuge at $1500 \times g$ for 2 min. Carefully remove the supernatant. Repeat washing the resin three more times.

8. Add 0.2 ml of elution buffer to the resin and gently shake for 4 min. Centrifuge at $1500 \times g$ for 5 min. Carefully transfer the supernatant to a fresh tube. Repeat this step two more times.

9. Pool the supernatant and add 0.1 volume 3 M sodium acetate and 2.5 volumes of 100% chilled ethanol to precipitate the mRNA. Mix and place at –20°C overnight.

10. Centrifuge at $12,000 \times g$ for 15 min and briefly wash the mRNA pellet with 1 ml of 70% ethanol. Dry the pellet under vacuum for 15 min and dissolve the mRNA in 10 μl of TE buffer. Take 2 μl of the sample to measure the concentration and quality of the mRNA. Store at –70°C until use.

Reagents Needed

Solution A

         4 M Guanidinium thiocyanate
         25 mM Sodium citrate, pH 7.0
         0.5% Sarcosyl
         Sterile-filter and store in a dark bottle at room temperature up to 3 months

Solution B

         100 ml Solution A
         0.72 ml β-Mercaptoethanol
         Store at room temperature up to 1 month.

Sodium Acetate Buffer (pH 4.0)

         2 M Sodium acetate

General Molecular Biology Techniques 193

Adjust pH to 4.0 with 2 *N* acetic acid. Autoclave.

Sodium Acetate Solution

3 *M* Sodium acetate
Autoclave

Water-Saturated Phenol

Thaw crystals of phenol at 65°C in a water bath and mix 1 part of phenol and 1 part of sterile ddH$_2$O. Mix well and allow two phases to separate. Store at 4°C.

Caution: *Phenol is a dangerous reagent; gloves should be worn and a fume hood should be used.*

Chloroform:lsoamyl Alcohol (49:1)

98 ml Chloroform
2 ml Isoamyl alcohol
Mix and store at 4°C.

Ethanol

70% Ethanol: 70 ml of 100% ethanol and 30 ml ddH$_2$O
75% Ethanol: 75 ml of 100% ethanol and 25 ml ddH$_2$O
100% Ethanol: store at –20°C.

20% SDS

20 g SDS (Sodium dodecyl sulfate) in 100 ml ddH$_2$O

0.1 N NaOH

0.4 g NaOH in 100 ml ddH$_2$O

RNA Extraction Solution

3 *M* LiC1(126 g)
6 *M* Urea (360 g)
Dissolve LiCl prior to adding urea. Adjust the volume to 1 liter with ddH$_2$O and then sterile-filter.

RNA Buffer

10 m*M* Tris-HC1, pH 7.5
1 m*M* EDTA, pH 8.0
0.2% SDS

PCR Protocols in Molecular Toxicology

Binding Buffer

10 mM Tris-HC1, pH 7.5
0.5 M NaCl
1 mM EDTA
0.5% SDS

Loading Buffer

20 mM Tris-HC1, pH 7.5
1 M NaCl
2 mM EDTA
0.2% SDS

Wash Buffer

10 mM Tris-HC1, pH 7.5
100 mM NaCl
1 mM EDTA
Autoclave

Elution Buffer

10 mM Tris-HC1, pH 7.5
1 mM EDTA

TE Buffer

10 mM Tris-HC1, pH 8.0
1 mM EDTA

Homogenization Buffer

50 mM NaCl
50 mM Tris-HC1, pH 7.5
5 mM EDTA, pH 8.0
0.5% SDS
200 µg/ml Proteinase K (from a stock solution of 20 mg/ml)

LiCl Solution

8 M LiCl Dissolved in distilled water and autoclaved

CsCl/EDTA Solution

5.7 M CsCl, 96.0 g of solid CsCl
Dissolve in 90 ml of 0.01 M EDTA, pH 7.5.
Add DEPC to a final concentration of 0.1%.

General Molecular Biology Techniques   **195**

Allow the solution to stand for 1 h.

Autoclave for 20 min at 15 psi in liquid cycle.

When it has cooled to room temperature, adjust the volume to 100 ml with DEPC-treated water.

Caution: *DEPC is a carcinogen and should be handled with care. Gloves should be worn when working with this reagent.[4]*

C.   Measurement of RNA

This procedure is based on reference 1.

Protocol

1. Turn on the ultraviolet (UV) spectrophotometer and set the wavelength to 260 and 280 nm according to the instructions. Some spectrophotometers (e.g., UV 160U, Shimadzu) contain a computer unit that can automatically and simultaneously measure RNA at wavelengths of 260 and 280 nm, and calculate and display RNA concentration together with the ratio of A_{260}/A_{280} numbers on the computer screen. If such a spectrophotometer is not available, RNA concentration can be measured by other, relatively simple UV spectrophotometers. The disadvantages are that the RNA first has to be measured and recorded at 260 nm and then at 280 nm, and that the RNA concentration and the ratio of A_{260}/A_{280} have to be calculated manually.

2. Set up a reference using blank solution. Depending on the RNA sample, add 1 ml of TE buffer (pH 8.0) or ddH_2O to a clean cuvette or to each of two cuvettes (one half to three quarters full), depending on whether one or two cells are available in the spectrophotometer. Insert the cuvette(s) into cuvette holder(s) in the sample compartment with the optical (clear) sides of the cuvette(s) facing the light path. Close the sample compartment cover and adjust the number to 0.000 (either manually or by pressing the Auto Zero button, depending on the specific spectrophotometer).

Caution: *Gloves should be worn when handling cuvettes. Cuvettes should be rinsed with 95% ethanol followed by ddH_2O, and wiped dry with Kimwipe paper prior to reuse.*

3. In a clean cuvette, appropriately dilute the RNA sample to be measured in blank solution to a total volume of 1 ml. For example, for 25 μl of RNA sample, the blank solution should be 975 μl. Wrap the cuvette in a piece of Parafilm and mix well by inverting the cuvette two to three times.

4. Insert the sample cuvette and read the absorbance of the sample cuvette against the blank cuvette according to the spectrophotometer instructions. If only one cell is available, remove the reference cuvette after adjusting the number to 0.000 and insert the sample cuvette. After measuring RNA sample(s) at 260 and 280

nm, respectively, calculate the ratio of A_{260}/A_{280} and concentration for each RNA sample. A pure RNA should have a A_{260}/A_{280} ratio of 1.85 to 2.0. The concentration of an RNA sample can be manually calculated as follows:

$$\text{Total RNA } (\mu g/ml) = A_{260} \times 40 \; \mu g/ml \times \text{dilution factor}$$

$$\text{Poly (A)}^+ \text{ RNA } (\mu g/ml) = A_{260} \times 42 \; \mu g/ml \times \text{dilution factor}$$

Note: *The dilution factor = (total volume/aliquot measured). For example, adding a 5 μl aliquot to 995 μl ddH₂O results in a dilution factor of 200.*

V. Subcloning the DNA Fragment of Interest

There are at least four advantages of subcloning a DNA fragment of interest as opposed to keeping the sample as a PCR product. First, the DNA fragment can be amplified up to 300-fold using a high copy number of plasmids that replicate in short-life cycle *E. coli*. Second, plasmids used for subcloning are designed to contain SP6, T7, or T3 promoters upstream from the polycloning sites, thus allowing one to prepare sense RNA or antisense RNA of the insert for analysis. Third, the merit of having an appropriate primer corresponding to SP6, T7, or T3 allows one to sequence the insert of interest on both strands in opposite directions. In addition, a known DNA sequence, such as cDNA or a genomic gene, can be ligated to appropriate vectors for gene transfer and expression analysis. For these purposes, the recombinant vectors (usually plasmids) may need to be subcloned. Therefore, subcloning is currently an essential technique used in molecular biology studies. The present section describes the detailed protocol for subcloning the DNA fragment, gene, or cDNA of interest, and selection of transformants.

A. Restriction Enzyme Digestion of Vector and DNA Insert for Subcloning

This procedure is based on reference 2.

Several commercial plasmids are available for cloning (see Appendix I and II for a list of suppliers). Selection of a particular plasmid vector depends on many different factors. Generally speaking, a standard plasmid for cloning should have the following necessary characteristics: 1) a polycloning site for the insertion of the foreign DNA of interest; 2) SP6, T7, or T3, or equivalent promoters upstream from the polylinker site located in opposite directions in order to express the DNA insert for sense RNA, antisense RNA, or protein analysis; 3) the origin of replication for the duplication of the recombinant

General Molecular Biology Techniques   **197**

plasmid in the host cell; 4) a selectable marker gene such as Amp^r for antibiotic selections of transformants; and 5) a selectable marker gene such as the lacZ gene containing the polycloning site for color (e.g., blue-white) screening of interesting bacterial colonies that contain the recombinant plasmids.

Protocol A — Preparation of Vectors

1. Set up, on ice, a standard single-restriction enzyme digestion as follows:
    Plasmid DNA (10 μg)
    10X Appropriate restriction enzyme buffer (10 μl)
    1 mg/ml acetylated BSA (optional) (10 μl)
    Appropriate restriction enzyme (3.3 units/μg DNA)
    Add ddH$_2$O to a final volume of 100 μl.

Notes: *The restriction enzyme used for vector and insert DNA digestions should be the same in order to ensure optimal ligation. For directional cloning, the plasmid and insert DNA should be digested using two different restriction enzymes. The double-enzyme digestion of DNA may be set up as a single reaction at the same time or be carried out as two single-enzyme digestions at different times. For double-restriction enzyme digestions, the appropriate 10X buffer containing a higher NaCl concentration than the other buffer may be chosen for the double enzyme digestion buffer.*

Set up, on ice, the double-restriction enzyme reaction as follows:
Plasmid DNA (10 μg)
10X Appropriate restriction enzyme buffer (10 μl)
1 mg/ml acetylated BSA (optional) (10 μl)
Appropriate restriction enzyme A (3.3 units/μg DNA)
Appropriate restriction enzyme B (3.3 units/μg DNA)
Add ddH$_2$O to a final volume of 100 μl.

2. Incubate at an appropriate temperature (e.g., 37°C) for 2 to 3 h. For single-enzyme-digested DNA, proceed to Step 3. For double-enzyme-digested DNA, proceed to Step 5. Run a small aliquot (10 μl) on a 1% agarose gel and compare to undigested vector. A partially digested enzyme will cause very large background in subsequent experiments. If the vector is not fully linearized, incubate overnight at 37°C.

3. Carry out the calf intestinal alkaline phosphatase (CIAP) treatment by adding the following directly to the single-enzyme-digested DNA sample (90 μl).
    10X CIAP buffer (15 μl)
    CIAP diluted in 10X CIAP buffer (0.01 unit/pmol ends)
    Add ddH$_2$O to a final volume of 150 μl.

198   PCR Protocols in Molecular Toxicology

Note: *CIAP and 10X CIAP should be kept at 4°C. CIAP treatment should*
          be set up at 0°C. Calculation of the amount of ends is as follows:
          There is 9 µg digested DNA left after taking 1 µg of 10 µl digested
          DNA for checking on agarose gel. If the vector is 3.2 Kb, the amount
          of ends can be calculated by the formula below:

$$\text{pmol ends} = (\text{amount of DNA})/(\text{bp} \times 660/\text{base pair}) \times 2$$

$$= 9\,\mu g/(3200 \times 660) \times 2$$

$$= 8.4 \times 10^{-6} = 8.4\,\text{pmol ends}$$

4.   Incubate at 37°C for 1 h and add 2 µl of 0.5 M EDTA buffer (pH 8.0) to stop
     the reaction. Extract with 1 volume of TE-saturated phenol/chloroform. Mix well
     by vortexing for 1 min and centrifuge at $12,000 \times g$ for 5 min at room temperature.

5.   Carefully transfer the top, aqueous phase to a fresh tube and add 1 volume of
     chloroform:isoamyl alcohol (24:1) to the supernatant. Mix well and centrifuge
     as in Step 5.

6.   Carefully transfer the upper, aqueous phase to a fresh tube and add 0.1 volume
     of 3 M sodium acetate buffer (pH 5.2) or 0.5 volume of 7.5 M ammonium acetate
     to the supernatant. Briefly mix and add 2.5 volumes of chilled 100% ethanol to
     the supernatant. Allow to precipitate at –70°C for 1 h or at –20°C for 2 h.

7.   Centrifuge at $12,000 \times g$ for 10 min and carefully decant the supernatant. Briefly
     rinse the DNA pellet with 1 ml of 70% ethanol and dry the pellet under vacuum
     for 20 min. Dissolve the DNA pellet in 20 to 40 µl ddH$_2$O. Take 4 µl of the
     sample to measure the concentration of the DNA at 260 nm. Store the sample
     at –20°C until use.

Protocol B — Preparation of Insert DNA

1.   Purify insert DNA from an agarose gel as described below

Note: *Insert DNA whose size is <4 Kb is easier for successful subcloning*
          than DNA whose size is 4 to 12 Kb.

2.   Carry out restriction enzyme digestion, purification, and precipitation the same
     as for vector DNA (Steps 1 through 7 in Protocol A).

Reagents Needed

Appropriate Enzymes

10X appropriate restriction enzyme buffer

1% agarose mini-gel

General Molecular Biology Techniques   **199**

TE-saturated phenol/chloroform

Chloroform:isoamyl alcohol (24:1)

3 M sodium acetate buffer, pH 5.2

7.5 M ammonium acetate

Ethanol (100%, 70%)

0.5 M EDTA, pH 8.0

Calf intestinal alkaline phosphatase (CIAP)

TE buffer

10X CIAP Buffer
>   0.5 M Tris-HCl, pH 9.0
>   10 mM MgCl$_2$
>   1 mM ZnCl$_2$
>   10 mM Spermidine

B.   Ligation of Plasmid Vector and Insert DNA

To achieve optimal ligation, the ratio of vector to insert DNA (1:1, 1:2, 1:3, and 3:1 molar ratios) should be optimized by using a small-scale reaction. The following reaction is standard for the ligation of a 3.2 Kb plasmid vector and a 3.0 Kb insert DNA.

Protocol

1. Calculate the molar weights of vector and insert DNA:
    1 mole plasmid vector = $3.2 \times 1000 \times 660 = 2.112 \times 10^6$ g
    1 mole insert DNA = $3 \times 1000 \times 660 = 1.98 \times 10^6$ g
2. Calculate the molar ratio of vector to insert DNA using Table 6.2.
3. Set up the ligations in Table 6.3 on ice.

Note: The restriction enzyme-digested plasmid (vector) and insert DNA should be dissolved in ddH$_2$O (nuclease free) at 0.5 to 1.0 μg/μl. If

PCR Protocols in Molecular Toxicology

TABLE 6.2
Calculation of Molar Ratios

	Amount of DNA (µg)	
Vector DNA:Insert	DNA Vector	Insert
1:1	1	0.792
1:2	1	1.584
1:3	1	2.376
3:1	1	0.264

the DNA is less than 0.4 µg/µl it should be precipitated so as to dissolve at about 1 µg/µl.

4. Incubate the reactions at 4°C for 12 to 24 h, or 16°C for 4 to 6 h, or at room temperature (22 to 25°C) for 1 to 2 h.

Note: *After the ligations are completed at the above temperatures, the mixture can be stored at 4°C until use.*

5. (Optional) Check the efficiency of the ligations by 1% agarose electrophoresis. When the electrophoresis is complete, photograph the gel stained with EtBr under UV light. As compared with unligated vector or insert DNA, high-efficiency ligation should make it possible to visualize if the vector and insert DNA are ligated to each other and show strong band(s) with molecular weight shifts compared to the vector and insert DNA sizes. By comparing the efficiency of ligations using different molar ratios, the optimal conditions can be determined with ease. These can be used as a guide for subsequent ligation.

6. If the ligation appears to have worked efficiently, proceed to the transformation reactions.

C. Bacterial Transformation

1. Prepare the LB medium and LB plates as described previously. This should be done before ligation.

2. Prepare competent cells as follows. This should be completed before ligation.

TABLE 6.3
Components of Ligation Reactions

Components	Ligation reactions			
	1 (1:1)	2 (1:2)	3(1:3)	4 (3:1)
Plasmid DNA as vector (µg)	1	1	1	1
Insert DNA (µg)	0.792	1.584	2.376	0.244
10X Ligase buffer (µl)	1	1	1	1
T4 DNA ligase (Weiss units)	4	4	4	4
Add ddH$_2$O to (µl)	10	10	10	10

General Molecular Biology Techniques 201

Protocol A — Preparation of Competent Cells for CaCl₂ Transformation

1. Streak the appropriate *E. coli* strain (DH5α or JM109 for color screening) directly from a small amount of frozen stock stored at –70°C onto the surface of an LB plate using a sterile platinum wire loop. Invert the plate and incubate in a 37°C incubator for 12 to 16 h. Bacterial colonies will become visible.

2. Inoculate a well-isolated colony from the plate at Step 1 into 50 ml of LB medium supplemented with 0.5 ml of 20% maltose and 0.5 ml of 1 M MgSO₄ solution. Incubate at 37°C overnight, shaking at 200 to 250 rpm.

3. Add 0.5 ml of cells from Step 2 to 100 ml of LB medium containing 1 ml of 20% maltose and 1 ml of 1 M MgSO₄ solution. Prepare four 100-ml cell cultures. Incubate at 37°C, shaking at 160 rpm, until the A_{600} reaches 0.45 to 0.6. It usually takes 2 to 5 h.

4. Chill the cells in ice water for 2 h and centrifuge at 3000 × g for 15 min at 4°C.

5. Resuspend the cells in 20 ml of ice-cold trituration buffer and dilute to 400 ml with the same buffer.

6. Incubate the cells on ice for 45 to 60 min.

7. Centrifuge at 2000 × g for 10 min at 4°C and gently resuspend the cells in 40 ml of ice-cold trituration buffer.

8. Add glycerol dropwise with gentle swirling to the cell solution to final concentration of 15% (v/v). Aliquot the cells at 0.2 ml per tube, freeze on dry ice, and then store at –70°C until use.

Protocol B — Preparation of Competent Cells for Heat Shock Transformation

1. Carry out Steps 1 through 4 in Protocol A.

2. Extensively wash the cells with 100 ml distilled water or low-salt buffer to reduce the ionic strength of the cell suspension.

3. Centrifuge at 2000 × g for 10 min at 4°C and carefully decant the supernatant.

4. Repeat Steps 2 and 3 twice.

5. Resuspend the cells in 200 ml of low-salt buffer or distilled water. Add glycerol dropwise with gentle swirling to 10% (v/v). Dispense the cell suspension into 20 µl per tube aliquots at approximately 3 × 10⁹ cells/ml. Freeze on dry ice and then store at –70°C until use.

D. Transformation Using Heat Shock Method

Protocol

For heat-shock transformation of *E. coli* follow the procedures listed below. Each bacterial strain has different optimal transformation conditions. The

202   PCR Protocols in Molecular Toxicology

appropriate conditions for DH5α cells (Gibco BRL), a good, standard efficiency strain that allows for blue-white screening, are given.

1. Thaw competent *E. coli* on ice.
2. Add 10 μl ligation reaction to 50 μl *E. coli* and let sit on ice for 30 min.
3. Place in 37°C water for 30 sec.
4. Put tubes back on ice for 2 min.
5. Add 1 mL LB or SOC media.
6. Shake tubes (220 rpm) at 37°C for 1 h.
7. Spin briefly in a microfuge, remove supernatant and *gently* resuspend in 100 μl LB media.
8. Spread 90 μl and 10 μl on each of two LB agar plates (with IPTG and X-Gal if blue-white screening is performed).
9. Grow inverted at 37°C overnight.

E.   Transformation Using the CaCl$_2$ Method

Protocol

1. Thaw three aliquots of 0.2 ml of frozen CaCl$_2$-treated competent cells on ice.
2. Add 3 μl of frozen-thawed DMSO to every 0.2-ml aliquot, mix, and add recombinant plasmid DNA as shown in Table 6.4.
3. Incubate on ice for 30 min.
4. Heat shock at 42°C for 2 min and place on ice for 1 min (optional).
5. Transfer the cell suspension to sterile culture tubes and add 2 ml of LB medium containing 20 μl of 20% maltose and 20 μl of 1 M MgSO$_4$ solution. Incubate at 37°C for 1 to 2 h with shaking at 140 rpm to recover the cells.
6. Add 50 to 150 μl of the culture per plate to the centers of LB plates containing 50 μg/ml ampicillin, 0.5 mM IPTG, and 40 μg/ml X-Gal. Quickly spread the cells over the entire surface of the LB plates using a sterile, bent glass rod.

Note: Transformations using different amounts of DNA at Step 2 should be plated at the same volume in order to determine the optimal conditions.

F.   Selection of Transformants Containing Recombinant Plasmids

Protocol

1. Invert all the plates prepared in Section V.E and V.G and incubate in a 37°C incubator for 12 to 16 h until colonies are visible.

General Molecular Biology Techniques

TABLE 6.4
Aliquot Components

Components	1	2	3
Cells (µl)	20	20	20
DMSO (µl)	3	3	3
DNA (µl)	1 (15 ng)	1 (100 ng)	1 (200 ng)

2. Chill the plates at 4°C for 1 h to maximally expose the blue colonies that may be not obvious when they are first taken from the incubator.

Notes: *Blue colonies contain nonrecombinant plasmid. β-Galactosidase expressed by the lacZ gene hydrolyzes X-Gal, forming a blue color. White colonies are supposed to bear recombinant plasmid in which foreign DNA was inserted at the polycloning site in the lacZ gene. The interrupted lacZ gene cannot express β-galactosidase activity. Therefore, the colonies are white.*

3. Inoculate individual white colonies into 5 ml of LB medium. Incubate at 37°C overnight with shaking at 160 rpm.

Note: *To verify white colonies, at least 20 individual colonies should be analyzed.*

4. Isolate plasmids as described in Section III.
5. Digest the plasmids with the same restriction enzyme(s) digestion as used for subcloning of the DNA insert of interest.
6. Carry out electrophoresis as previously described.
7. Photograph and verify the sizes of the vector and insert DNA as compared with unligated vector and insert DNA.
8. Inoculate 0.5 ml of the verified white colony cells into 100 ml of LB medium containing 50 µg/ml ampicillin and 1 ml of 1 M MgSO$_4$ solution. Incubate at 37°C overnight while shaking at 160 rpm.
9. Aliquot 1 ml of the culture to microfuge tubes and add glycerol dropwise to 15% (w/v). Freeze on dry ice and store at −70°C for further use. Carry out isolation and purification of the recombinant plasmids as described previously.

Reagents Needed

LB (Luria-Bertaini) Medium

Bacto-tryptone (10 g)
Bacto-yeast extract (5 g)
NaCl (5 g)
Adjust the pH to 7.5 with 2 N NaOH solution and autoclave.
When it has cooled, store at 4°C until use. Make 4 liters.

204 PCR Protocols in Molecular Toxicology

LB Plates

Add 15 g agar per liter unautoclaved LB medium. Adjust the pH to 7.5 with 2 N NaOH solution. Autoclave. When it has cooled to 50 to 55°C, add 50 µg/ml ampicillin, 0.5 mM IPTG, and 40 µg/ml X-Gal. (IPTG and X-Gal are optional). Mix well and pour into culture plates (30 to 35 ml per plate) in a sterile laminar flow hood. Cover the plates and allow to harden for 1 h. Let the plates set at room temperature for two days before use. The plates can be placed at room temperature for up to 10 days, or wrapped and stored at 4°C for up to 1 month. The plates should be placed at room temperature prior to being used.

Trituration Buffer

0.1 M CaCl$_2$
70 mM MgCl$_2$
40 mM Sodium acetate, pH 5.5
Freshly prepare and sterile-filter.

0.1 M IPTG Solution

1.2 g IPTG in 50 ml ddH$_2$O
Filter-sterilize and store at 4°C.

X-Gal Stock Solution

50 mg/ml Stock in N,N'-dimethylformamide

VI. Chloroform:Phenol Extraction of DNA

This discussion is based on reference 1.

1. To the DNA, add 1 volume TE-buffered phenol/chloroform (1:1, v/v), vortex for 1 minute and centrifuge for 2 minutes at 12,000 × g.

2. Carefully remove the top, aqueous layer and transfer to a fresh tube. Add 0.5 volume of 7.5 M ammonium acetate and 2 volumes chilled 100% ethanol. Vortex briefly and precipitate at –70°C for 30 min.

3. Centrifuge at 12,000 × g for 10 minutes, decant the supernatant and briefly rinse the pellet with 1 ml 70% ethanol. Dry the pellet for 15 minutes under vacuum and dissolve the DNA in an appropriate volume of ddH$_2$O.

4. Take 2 µl of the sample to measure the concentration of the DNA using UV spectroscopy. Estimate the amount of DNA present using the following formula:

$$\mu g/\mu l \text{ sample} = \text{Absorption at 260 nm} \times 0.04 \text{ } \mu g/\mu l \times \text{dilution factor}$$

General Molecular Biology Techniques

VII. Agarose Gel Electrophoresis of DNA

This section is based on reference 1.

A. General Considerations

Agarose gel electrophoresis is a standard method used to separate, identify, and purify DNA fragments including PCR products. Agarose is extracted from seaweed and is a linear polymer of D-galactose and L-galactose. When agarose is melted and then allowed to harden, it forms a matrix which serves as a molecular sieve to separate DNA fragments. For analysis of PCR products, we recommend a mixture of different agaroses, 3 parts low-melting to 1 part standard agarose (i.e., NuSieve 3:1, FMC). This gives excellent resolution of small products, plus has enough strength to make it easy to handle. The following factors should be considered for the rate at which DNA fragments migrate in an agarose gel.

1. Agarose concentration should be determined as follows:

   Gel percentage (w/v) Linear DNA separation range (Kb):

Standard Agarose

Percent (w/v)	kb resolved
0.6%	1–20
0.7%	0.8–10
1%	0.5–8
1.2%	0.4–6
1.4%	0.2–4

Gel percentage (w/v) Linear DNA separation range (bp):

3:1 Mixture Low Melting:Standard Agarose (i.e., NuSieve 3:1, FMC Products)

Percent (w/v)	bp resolved
2.0%	500–1000
3.0%	150–700
3.5%	100–450
4.0%	70–300

206   PCR Protocols in Molecular Toxicology

2. **The sizes of DNA fragments** — Linear duplex molecules travel through the gel matrix at a rate inversely proportional to the log of their molecular weight. The smaller the fragment, the faster it moves.

3. **DNA conformation** — DNA shape also influences the migration rate. For a DNA fragment with a particular size, the migration rate will be:

   Closed circular (supercoiled > slightly coiled) > linear > open circular

4. **Current applied** — The migration of DNA fragments is directly proportional to the voltage applied. Too high or too low a voltage is not recommended. The normal voltage should be 5 to 10 V/cm. The distance is referred to the length of the gel between the negative and the positive electrodes.

Protocol

1. Prepare DNA sample(s) for electrophoresis by adding the appropriate amount of 10X loading dye. The minimum amount of specific band to be detected is approximately 15 to 25 ng.

2. Thoroughly clean the appropriate gel apparatus by washing with detergent, completely removing the detergent mixture with tap water and rinsing with distilled water three to five times. Allow the apparatus to dry at room temperature.

3. Prepare an agarose mixture in a clean bottle or a beaker as follows:

	Components		
	Mini gel	**Midi gel**	**Big gel**
1X TBE or TAE buffer	40 ml	100 ml	220 ml
NuSieve Agarose (3% w/v)	1.2 g	3 g	6.6 g

Notes: *IX TBE or TAE buffer may be diluted from 10X TBE or 10X TAE stock solution with ddH$_2$O*

4. Slightly mix and melt the agarose by gently boiling in a microwave oven for 1 to 3 min depending on the gel volume. Alternatively, put a magnetic stir bar in the bottle or beaker and heat on a stirring hot plate, gently boiling until agarose dissolves. Gently mix and place at room temperature to cool to 50 to 60°C.

5. While the gel mixture is cooling, seal the air-dried gel tray at the two open ends with a tape or gasket and insert the comb. Add 10 µl of 10 mg/ml ethidium bromide (EtBr) to 100 ml of agarose gel solution (50 to 60°C), gently mix, and slowly pour into the assembled gel tray. Allow the gel to harden for 20 to 30 min at room temperature.

Caution: *EtBr is a mutagen and a potential carcinogen. Gloves should be worn when working with this material. The gel running buffer containing EtBr should be collected in a special container.[4]*

General Molecular Biology Techniques

207

> *Notes: EtBr is used to stain DNA or RNA molecules. It intercalates between the complementary strands of a double-strand DNA or in the regions of secondary structure in the case of ssDNA or RNA and fluoresces orange when illuminated with UV light. The merit of adding EtBr to the gel is that DNA bands can be stained and monitored with a UV lamp during electrophoresis. The drawback, however, is that running buffer and gel apparatus are contaminated with EtBr. An alternative way is to carry out electrophoresis without EtBr. The gel is then stained with EtBr for 10 to 30 min following electrophoresis.*

6. Carefully remove the comb and sealing tape or gasket from the gel tray. Place the gel tray in the electrophoresis tank and add enough 1X TBE or TAE buffer to the tank until the gel is covered to a depth of 1.5 to 2 mm above the gel.

> *Notes: The comb should be slowly and vertically removed from the gel, since any cracks inside the wells of the gel will cause leaking when the sample is loaded. The well-side of the gel must be placed at the negative pole end since the negatively charged DNA will migrate toward the positive pole. When the gel is covered with running buffer, each well should be flushed with the buffer using a small pipette tip to flush the buffer up and down inside the well several times. The purpose of doing this is to remove any potential bubbles that will adversely influence the loading of the samples and the electrophoresis.*

7. Prerun the gel at a constant voltage (5 to 10 V/cm) for 10 min, but this is optional.

8. Add 10X loading buffer to the DNA sample and DNA standard marker to a final concentration of 1X. Mix well. Carefully load the samples and one lane with a commercial DNA standard marker (0.2 to 2 µg per well).

9. Measure the length of the gel between the two electrodes and apply power to 5 to 10 V/cm. Allow the electrophoresis to run for an appropriate amount of time to get resolution of the products (usually 45 to 90 min).

10. Stop the electrophoresis of the gel and remove to observe under UV light. Photograph the gel with a Polaroid™ camera or equivalent.

> *Caution: Wear safety glasses and gloves for protection from UV light.*

B. Purifying DNA Fragments from Agarose Gels

1. Freeze-and-Squeeze Method

1. Resolve DNA fragments on an agarose gel as discussed above. Low melting agarose is recommended. Visualize the fragment of interest by ethidium bromide staining.

208 PCR Protocols in Molecular Toxicology

Note: *Short exposure to a long-wavelength UV transilluminator is recommended. This will reduce the amount of damage to DNA. Short-wavelength UV light can cause DNA strand breaks and decrease the ability to subclone the fragment.*

2. Cut and remove the DNA fragment using a clean razor blade and place in a microfuge tube. Remove as little of the gel as possible.
3. Add 2 volumes of TE buffer to the gel slices and completely melt the gel in a 65°C water bath.
4. Immediately place the melted gel solution in a –70°C freezer for 20 min.
5. Thaw the gel mixture and tap the tube vigorously.
6. Centrifuge at 10,000 × *g* for 5 min at room temperature.
7. Transfer the liquid phase to a fresh tube. Chloroform:phenol extract the DNA as discussed above.

2.   Elution from Wells of Agarose Gels

1. Perform electrophoresis as described above, except fill the buffer reservoir with running buffer until only the edges of the agarose are submerged.
2. While monitoring with a UV light, electrophorese the DNA until the fragment of interest has separated from other products. Stop the electrophoresis and use a razor blade or spatula to cut a well directly in front of the appropriate band. Add 50 µl of buffer to the well.
3. Continue electrophoresis, while monitoring with UV light, until the band migrates into the well.
4. Stop the electrophoresis, transfer the buffer in the well to a fresh tube and continue with chloroform:phenol extraction as discussed above.

Reagents Needed

Ultrapure Agarose or Agarose Mixture

Gel Casting Tray

Gel Combs

DC Power Supply

10X TBE Buffer

600 ml ddH₂O
0.9 *M* Tris base (108 g)

General Molecular Biology Techniques

0.9 *M* Boric acid (55 g)
0.02 *M* EDTA (40 ml 0.5 *M* EDTA, pH 8.0)
Dissolve well after each addition. Add ddH$_2$O to 1 liter
Autoclave.

10X TAE Buffer

600 ml ddH$_2$O
0.4 *M* Tris-acetate (48.4 g Tris base, 11.42 ml glacial acetic
acid)
10 m*M* EDTA (20 ml 0.5 *M* EDTA, pH 8.0)
Dissolve or mix well after each addition. Add ddH$_2$O to 1 liter
Sterile-filter.

Ethidium Bromide (EtBr)

10 mg/ml in ddH$_2$O
Dissolve well and keep in a dark or brown bottle at 4°C.

5X Glycerol Loading Buffer

50% Glycerol
1 m*M* EDTA
0.25% Bromophenol blue
0.25% Xylene cyanol (optional)
Dissolve well and store at 4°C.

10X Ficoll Loading Buffer

30% Ficoll in TE buffer
0.25% Bromophenol blue
0.25% Xylene cyanol (optional)

VIII. Transfection of Mammalian Cells

There are several methods that may be used to transfect mammalian cells with
plasmid DNA including calcium phosphate coprecipitation, DEAE-Dextran,
and electroporation. The calcium phosphate procedure is the easiest to perform
and works well for reporter assays as discussed in Chapter 4 for a variety of
cell types. The following procedure assumes that the conditions for growth
and maintenance of your mammalian cell line have been optimized.

1. Plate the cells the day before the transfection experiment. The cells should be
    approximately 80% confluent on the day of transfection.

Note: *As a general guideline, the cells should be plated at approximately 5.5×10^5 cells per 60 mm dish, 1.5×10^6 cells per 100 mm dish, or 5×10^4 cells per 24-well dish. Scale the number of cells proportionally to the growth area of the plate.*

2. Three hours prior to transfection remove the media from the cells and replace with fresh growth media.

3. For each transfection, prepare the following in sterile tubes. Use tubes per plate. In the first tube, add the DNA and water to the tube, mix well, then add the 2 M CaCl$_2$. In the second tube add the 2X HBS.

Tube 1	Per 60 mm dish	Per 100 mm dish
Plasmid DNA*	10 μg	20 μg
2 M CaCl$_2$	37 μl	62 μl
Sterile ddH$_2$O	to 0.3 ml final	to 0.5 ml final

Tube 2		
2X HBS	0.3 ml	0.5 ml

* The amount of plasmid may require optimization. Also, make sure the plasmid is pure (we generally perform two chloroform:phenol extractions) and is resuspended in sterile ddH$_2$O.

4. In the tissue culture hood, *gently* vortex the tube containing the 2X HBS solution. Continue to vortex while adding the contents of tube 1 (dropwise). The resulting solution should look slightly opaque. Incubate the solution at room temperature for 30 min.

5. Vortex the solution immediately prior to adding it to the cells. Add the solution dropwise to the plates and swirl to distribute evenly. Return the plates to a 37°C CO$_2$/air incubator.

6. (Optional Steps 6 through 9). A glycerol shock 4 to 16 h after transfection may improve efficiency of DNA uptake. Prepare fresh glycerol shock solution in 1X HBS and warm to 37°C, along with the growth media and wash solution (1X sterile PBS).

7. Wash the cells once with PBS (5 ml for 60 mm or 10 ml for 100 mm plate)

8. Add 2 ml (60 mm) or 3 ml (100 mm) glycerol shock solution per plate. Incubate 2 min at room temperature.

9. Remove the glycerol shock solution and rinse twice with PBS as stated in Step 7.

10. Add growth media and place in 37°C CO$_2$/air incubator.

11. Change media 4 to 16 h after transfection.

General Molecular Biology Techniques

12. In general, cells may be harvested 48 to 72 hours after transfection for performing reporter assays as discussed in Chapter 4.

Reagents Needed

2X HBS (HEPES buffered saline)
50 mM HEPES, pH 7.1
280 mM NaCl
1.5 mM NaCl
1.5 mM Na$_2$HPO$_4$
The final pH should be 7.1

PBS 1X (sterile filter)
Per liter
0.2 g KCl
8.0 g NaCl
0.2 g KH$_2$PO$_4$
1.15 g Na$_2$HPO$_4$
Adjust pH to 7.4 with 1 N NaOH or 1 N HCl

Glycerol Shock Solution
Add sterile glycerol to 1X HBS to a final concentration of 15% (v/v)

References

1. **Kaufman, P.B., Wu, W., Kim, D., and Cseke, L.J.,** in *Handbook of Molecular and Cellular Methods in Biology and Medicine*, Kaufman et al., Eds., CRC Press, Boca Raton, FL, 1995.
2. **Sambrook, J., Fritsch, E.F., and Maniatis, T.,** *Molecular Cloning, A Laboratory Manual*, 2nd Ed., Cold Spring Harbor Press, Cold Spring Harbor, NY, 1989.
3. **Chomczynski, P. and Sacchi, N.,** Single step method for RNA isolation by acid guanidinium-thiocyanate-phenol-chloroform extraction, *Anal. Biochem.*, 162, 156, 1987.
4. **Lunn, G. and Sansone, E.R.,** Ethidium bromide: destruction and decontamination of solutions, *Anal. Biochem.*, 162, 453, 1987.

Appendix I

List of Suppliers

DNA Thermal Cyclers
The Perkin-Elmer Corporation
761 Main Avenue
Norwalk, CT 06859-0001
1-800-762-4000

MJ Research, Inc.
149 Grove Street
Watertown, MA 02172
1-800-729-2165

Ericomp
10055 Barnes Canyon Road
Suite G
San Diego, CA 92121

Reagents
(Taq DNA polymerase,
 dNTPs, reverse transcriptase,
 restriction enzymes, etc.)

Amersham North America
2636 South Clearbrook Drive
Arlington Heights
Illinois 60005, USA
1-800-323-9750

CLONTECH Laboratories, Inc.
1020 East Meadow Circle
Palo Alto, CA 94303-4230
1-800-662-CLON

Invitrogen Corporation
3985 B Sorrento Valley Blvd.
San Diego, CA 92121
1-800-955-6288

New England Biolabs, Inc.
32 Tozer Road
Beverly, MA 01915-5054
1-800-632-5227

Novagen, Inc.
597 Science Drive
Madison, WI 53711
1-800-207-0144

The Perkin-Elmer Corporation
761 Main Avenue
Norwalk, Connecticut 06859-0001
1-800-762-4000

Pharmacia Biotech AB
S-751 82 Uppsala, Sweden
Tel 46 (0)18 16 50 00

Promega Corporation Headquarters
2800 Woods Hollow Road
Madison, WI 53711
1-800-356-9526

Sigma Chemical Company
P.O. Box 14508
St. Louis, MO 63178 USA
800-325-3010

United States Biochemical Corp.
P.O. Box 22400
Cleveland, OH 44122

Worthington Biochemical Corporation
450 Halls Mills Road
Freehold, NJ 07728-9931
1-800-445-9603

Oligonucleotide Synthesis
Genosys Biotechnologies, Inc.
1442 Lake Front Circle, Suite 185
The Woodlands, TX 77380-3600
1-713-363-3693, 1-800-234-5362

Operon Technologies, Inc.
1000 Atlantic Ave., Suite 108
Alameda, CA 94501
1-800-688-2248

Ransom Hill Bioscience, inc.
P.O. Box 219
Ramona, CA 92065
619-789-9483

Research Genetics
US/Canada 800-533-4363,
World Wide Phone: 205-533-4363
UK: 0-800-89-1393, FAX: 205-536-9016
2130 Memorial Pkwy., SW
  Huntsville, AL 35801

General Chemicals
(Buffer components, ethidium
  bromide, Ficoll, bromophenol
  blue, mineral oil, etc.)

Sigma Chemical Company
P.O. Box 14508
St. Louis, MO 63178 USA
800-325-3010

Fisher Scientific
Headquarters
711 Forbes Avenue
Pittsburgh, PA 15219-4785
1-412-562-8300

Continental Laboratory Products Inc.
  (CLP) 800-456-7741
Midwest Scientific Telephone
  800-227-9997

Agarose and Purification Products
(For DNA resolution and
  purification)

AMRESCO
(800)829-2805
Supplied by:
Continental Laboratory Products Inc.
  (CLP) 800-456-7741
Midwest Scientific Telephone
  800-227-9997

Amicon, Inc.
72 Cherry Hill Drive
Beverly, MA 01915
508-777-3622

FMC Bioproducts
5 Maple St.
Rockland, ME 04841
1-800-438-6670

List of Suppliers

Millipore Corporation,
80 Ashby Road,
Bedford MA 01730
1-800-645-5476

Primer Design

DNASTAR
1228 South Park Street
Madison, Wisconsin 53715 USA
Phone: USA 608-258-7420

Premier Biosoft International
3786 Corina Way
Palo Alto, CA 95303
1-415-856-2703

Appendix II

Companies, Online Catalogs and Internet Resources

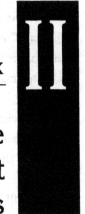

Company	Internet Address
5 prime -> 3 prime	http://www.5prime.com
Ambion, Inc.	http://www.ambion.com
Amersham International	http://www.amersham.com
Amicon	http://www.amicon.com
Beckman Instruments	http://www.beckman.com
Boehringer Mannheim Biochemicals	http://biochem.boehringer.com
Clontech	http://www.clontech.com
DNAStar	http://www.dnastar.com
Dupont NEN	http://www.nenlifesci.com
Eppendorf	http://www.eppendorf.com/eppendrf
EuGene Primer Design Software	http://www.daniben.com
Fisher Scientific	http://www.fisher1.com
FMC BioProducts	http://www.bioproducts.com
Gelman Sciences, Inc	http://argus-nc.com/Gelman/Gelman.html
Genosys Biotechnologies, Inc	http://www.genosys.com
Hitachi Software	http://www.hitsoft.com

0-8493-3344-X/98/$0.00+$.50
© 1998 by CRC Press LLC

Hybaid	http://www.hybaid.co.uk
Invitrogen	http://www.invitrogen.com
Life Technologies (Gibco/BRL)	http://www.lifetech.com
Millipore Corporation	http://www.millipore.com
National Instruments	http://webserver.natinst.com
New England Biolabs	http://vent.neb.com
Novagen	http://www.novagen.com
Operon Technologies	http://operon.com
Perkin-Elmer	http://www.perkin-elmer.com
Pharmacia Biotech	http://www.biotech.pharmacia.se
Promega	http://www.promega.com
Ransom Hill Bioscience	http://www.ransomhill.com
Research Genetics	http://www.resgen.com
Sigma Chemical	http://www.sigma.sial.com
Worthington Biochemical Corporation	http://www.worthington-biochem.com

Indexes and Resources	Internet Address
General Biotechnology Indexes	http://www.cato.com/interweb/cato/biotech/bio-prot.html
Company Pages	http://www.atcg.com/aguide/comppage/comppage.htm
Biosupplynet	http://www.biosupplynet.com/bsn
BioTechniques	http://www.biotechniques.com
Pedro's BioMolecular Research Tools	http://www.public.iastate.edu/~pedro/research_tools.html
The National Center for Biotechnology Information	http://www.ncbi.nlm.nih.gov
PCR Applications Manual	http://biochem.boehringer-mannheim.com/prod_inf/manuals/pcr_man/pcr_toc.html
The PCR Primers Database Home Page	http://www.ebi.ac.uk/primers_home.html

Index

A

Absorbance unit ratio, 74, 75
N-Acetyltranferase (NAT), 164
N-Acetyltransferase 2 (NAT2), 164, 167–172, 175
Acid citrate dextrose solution (ACD), 179, 182
Acrylamide, 148, 149
Actin, 44
β-Actin, 82
Additives, 30, 37–38. *See also* DMSO; Formamide; Glycerol; PEG; Perfect Match; Spermidine
Aerosol barrier tips, 60, 65
Agarose, suppliers, 214–215
Agarose gel electrophoresis of DNA, 205–209
Agar plate, growth of cloned fragments in DD PCR, 100, 102
Alkaline lysis, isolation of plasmid DNA by, 183–186
Allele-specific PCR, 164–165, 166
Alu I, 171, 175
α-Amanitin, 90
Ambion, Inc., 217
Amersham, 113, 213, 217
Amicon, Inc., 214, 217
Amino acid codons, 132
Ammonium acetate, 123, 180, 199
Ammonium persulfate, 149
Ammonium sulfate, 174
Ampicillin, 111, 183, 184, 203
Amplification
across an intron, 50–52
in cycle-based quantitative RT-PCR, 78–81
in differential display PCR, 101
of a dilution series of rcRNA, 60–63
of DNA pool, 149–150
internal standard, 46–47, 49–50, 51–52, 77
in Liang and Pardee method, 106–107
low-stringency, 48–50
rapid, of cDNA ends, 101, 122, 134–139, 144–145
in *in situ* RT-PCR, 87–88
in Sokolov and Prockop method, 108–109
Amplification buffer, 115
Amplification efficiency, 4–6
internal standard *vs.* target, 63
tube-to-tube variability, 44, 63, 77. *See also* Internal standard
yield *vs.* cycle number, 77
Amplification mix, 115
AmpliWax beads, 33
Amp^r gene, 197
AMRESCO, 214
AMV reverse transcriptase, 61, 128
in competitive quantitative RT-PCR procedure, 66
in reporter gene analysis, 92
Anchored PCR, 122
Annealing, basic considerations, 29–30
Annealing temperature. *See also* Thermocycle programs
basic cloning by RT-PCR, 129
construction of wild-type plasmid, 56
cycle-based quantitative RT-PCR, 81
direct sequencing by PCR, 156
generation of wild-type plasmid, 58, 59
hot start, 62, 68, 73

219

internal standard amplification, 46, 49, 52

library screening, 141, 143, 145

multiplex PCR for genotyping, 174

NAT2 genotyping, 170

on OLIGO software, 23, 24, 32

optimization experiment, 32–33

PCR amplification, 106, 107

PCR clone check, 154

on PRIMER software, 26

RACE, 136, 137, 139

selection and binding sites technique, 150, 151

semiquantitative RT-PCR, 85

standard RT-PCR, 62

Antibiotics

ampicillin, 111, 183, 184, 203

kanamycin, 111

YT plus antibiotic, 112

Antibodies, 88

cross-reacting, 132

monoclonal, 33

TaqStart, 33, 34, 35, 36, 38, 174

Antibody recognition sequences, 126

Apoptosis, 99

"Artifact"

in low-stringency amplification, 48

primer, methods to decrease. *See* Cold start; Hot start

Autoclave, 8

Autoradiography, 82, 107

B

Bacterial transformation, 200–201

Bacto-tryptone, 158, 185, 203

Bacto-yeast extract, 158, 185, 203

BamH I, 171, 175

Base changes, 164

Beckman Instruments, 217

Biosupplynet, 218

BioTechniques, 218

Bisacrylamide, 148, 149

Blood cells, extraction of genomic DNA from, 179

Blunt-end cloning, 123

Blunt-end enzyme, 123

Boehringer Mannheim Biochemicals, 88, 217

Boric acid, 209

Bovine serum albumin (BSA), 94, 95, 116, 155, 157, 174, 197

Bromophenol blue, 96, 115, 159, 160, 209

Browser software, 16

BSA. *See* Bovine serum albumin

Buffers

10X amplification, 115

chloroform/isoamyl alcohol, 184, 185, 186, 187, 193, 199

CIAP, 199

denaturation, 116, 182, 185

Ficoll loading, 96, 160, 209

first-strand, 108, 117

formamide loading, 115

forward exchange, 95, 157

gel shift 5X, 148, 158

glycerol loading, 209

Klenow 10X, 147

LB (Luria-Bertaini). *See* Luria-Bertaini buffer/medium

ligase, 95, 157

5X ligation, 111, 115

10X ligation, 56, 57, 125, 131

lysis, 181–182, 185

MMLV. *See* MMLV reverse transcriptase buffer

10X PCR

in basic cloning by RT-PCR, 66, 127, 128

in competitive quantitative RT-PCR procedure, 66

in competitive RT-PCR with standard curve, 70, 71, 72

in construction of a PCR cloning vector, 54

in construction of wild-type plasmid, 55

in cycle-based quantitative RT-PCR, 79, 80

in direct sequencing by PCR, 155, 157

in library screening, 140, 143, 144

in multiplex PCR for genotyping, 173, 174

in NAT2 genotyping, 169

in PCR clone check, 153

in PCR mutagenesis, 58, 59

in RACE, 135, 136, 137, 138

Index

in reporter gene analysis, 92, 93, 94–95
in selection and binding sites technique, 150, 151
in semiquantitative RT-PCR, 83, 84
in *in situ* RT-PCR, 87
in Sokolov and Prockop method, 108
in standard RT-PCR procedure, 60, 61
PCR Buffer II, 37
phenol/chloroform
in digestion of contaminating cDNA, 104
in direct sequencing by PCR, 158
in dot-blot differential hybridization, 117
in ligation reaction, 130
in mini-prep of plasmid DNA, 184, 186
in preparation of insert DNA, 199
in reporter gene analysis, 91
restriction enzyme, 123, 130, 154, 197, 198
RNA, 193
10X Rx, 30, 34, 36, 37, 46
sequencing, 159
6X, 115, 159
SM, 142, 144, 158
sodium acetate, 117, 189, 190, 192–193, 199
storage of, 8
suppliers of, 213–214
TAE, 206, 207, 209
tailing, 138
TaqStart, 35
TBE, 149, 206, 207, 208
TBS, 86, 88
TBS-MS, 88
TE
in direct sequencing by PCR, 157
in extraction of DNA, 179, 180, 204
in 5′ labeling of PCR primer, 78
in isolation of total RNA, 190
in measurement of RNA, 195
in preparation of insert DNA, 199
in preparation of plasmid DNA, 184, 185
in purification of mRNA, 194
in reporter gene analysis, 95

10X T4 polynucleotide kinase, 148, 157
transcription, 95, 157
trituration, 204

C

Calcium chloride, 204, 210
Calcium chloride transformation, 201, 202
Calcium phosphate coprecipitation, 209
Calf intestinal alkaline phosphatase (CIAP), 197, 198, 199
Carcinogenesis, 99, 164–165
Carcinogen metabolism polymorphisms, genotyping of, 164–165
cDNA
cloning, 110–112
contamination with, 103–104
rapid amplification of ends, 101, 122, 134–139, 144–145
reamplification of fragments, 109–110
synthesis
in differential display PCR, 101
Master Mix, 87
in *in situ* RT-PCR, 86–87
in Sokolov and Prockop method, 108
Cell cultures
extraction of genomic DNA from, 179–180
LiCl-urea and phenol-chloroform RNA extraction from, 188–189
rapid isolation of total RNA from, 187
Cellular differentiation, 99
Cellular injury, 99
Cesium chloride, 103, 189–190, 194
Chemical suppliers, 214
Chloramphenicol acetyl transferase (CAT), 91
Chloroform, 142
Chloroform/isoamyl alcohol buffer, 184, 185, 186, 187, 193, 199
Chloroform/phenol buffer. *See* Phenol/chloroform buffer
Chromosomal DNA. *See* cDNA
CIAP buffer, 199
CIAP (calf intestinal alkaline phosphatase), 197, 198, 199
Citric acid, 182

222 PCR Protocols in Molecular Toxicology

Clamp-restriction sites, 147
Clamp sequence, 126–127
Cloning. *See also* TA cloning
  differential display fragments, 110–112
  in differential display PCR, 100, 102
  by PCR, 121–160
  PCR clone check, 152–154
  of RACE products, 139
  by RT-PCR, 126–131
Cloning vector, construction of, 54–55,
    123–125
Clontech Laboratories, Inc., 33, 174, 213,
    217. *See also* TaqStart Antibody
Clorox, 8
Clothing, laboratory, 7
Coamplification. *See* Semiquantitative
    RT-PCR
Codons, redundancy of genetic code in,
    132
Cold start PCR, protocol, 62–63, 68, 73,
    81, 85, 129–130
Colony-PCR, confirmation of size of
    insert by, 112
Columns, oligo(dT)-cellulose, 190–195
Company Pages, 217–218
Competitive quantitative RT-PCR, 63–76,
    90
Competitive RT-PCR
  advantages, *vs.* cycle-based approach,
    63
  constant RNA with serial dilutions of
    internal standard, 65–69
  general, 64–69, 90
  with standard curve, 70–76
Computer databases, 9, 218
Computer files. *See* Electronic files
Contamination, 6
  with cDNA fragments, 103–104
  by internal standard, 60, 65, 70, 79
  in quantitation of hnRNA with genomic
    DNA, 89–90
  with RNase, 186
Continental Laboratory Products Inc., 214
Coolant, 8
Coprecipitation, calcium phosphate, 209
Cover slips, 86–87
Cresol red, 116
Crossover point
  in competitive RT-PCR, 64

  definition, 44
  plotting, 69
Cross-reacting antibodies, 132
Crystal Mount, 88
Cutting site, 127, 147, 164
Cuvettes, 195
Cycle-based quantitative RT-PCR, 76–82
Cycle number
  optimization experiment, 31–32, 35
  sizes of various genomes and copies per
    microgram, 31
  yield per. *See* Amplification efficiency

D

Databases, 9, 218
DD PCR. *See* Differential display PCR
DEAE-Dextran, 209
Decontamination, 8
Deep Vent, 21
Degenerate primer PCR, 131–134
Delta G values, 25
Denaturation, basic considerations, 29–30
Denaturation temperature
  basic cloning by RT-PCR, 129
  cycle-based quantitative RT-PCR,
    81
  direct sequencing by PCR, 156
  generation of wild-type plasmid, 56,
    58, 59
  hot start, 62, 68, 73
  internal standard amplification, 46, 49,
    52
  library screening, 141, 143, 145
  multiplex PCR for genotyping, 174
  NAT2 genotyping, 170
  PCR amplification, 106
  PCR clone check, 153
  RACE, 136, 137, 139
  selection and binding sites technique,
    150, 151
  semiquantitative RT-PCR, 85
  standard RT-PCR, 62
Denaturing buffer, 116, 182, 185
Denhardt's solution, 116
Densitometer, 68, 82
Deoxyribonucleotide triphosphate
    (dNTP), 2
  in hot start protocol, 35

Index

magnesium ion concentration and, 29, 30, 37

in oil-overlay thermocycler protocol, 31

in optimization experiments, 36, 37

DEPC. *See* Diethyl pyrocarbonate

Design
of laboratory, 6–8
of primers, 21–28

Detection, signal, 88. *See also* Quantitation detection

Detection limit, 6

DH5α cells, 57, 125, 131, 201, 202

Dideoxynucleotide chain termination methods, 154

Diethyl pyrocarbonate (DEPC)
to avoid RNase contamination, 186
in dot-blot differential hybridization, 117
in Liang and Pardee method, 103, 104, 105
in multiplex PCR genotyping of GSTM1 and GSTT1, 174
in purification of mRNA, 194–195
in rapid isolation of total RNA, 188
in Sokolov and Prockop method, 108

Differential display PCR (DD PCR), 99–117
cloning fragments from, 109–112
confirmation of altered expression with, 113–117
kits or products for, 103

Digitization of image, 68

Digoxigenin Detection Kit, 88

Digoxigenin (DIG), 87, 88, 107

Dilution screening, 140–142

Dilution series
competitive quantitative RT-PCR with, 65–68
internal standard, calculation of, 65
of rcRNA, amplification of, 60–63

Direct sequencing by PCR, 154–160

Dithiothreitol, 116, 117

Diversified Biotech, 107

DMSO, 26, 37, 136, 138, 202

DNA
amount of, calculation, 181, 200
conformation and migration rate, 206
electrophoresis of, 205–209

isolation and purification from animals, 179–182

isolation and purification of plasmid, 182–186

PCR product, amount, 55, 76, 125, 130

phenol/chloroform extraction of, 204

sample used for optimization, 31

storage of, 8

DNA amplification. *See* Amplification

DNA DataBank of Japan (DDBJ), 10

DNA enhancer regions, 43

DNA fragments
cloning, 110–112
false-positive, 103
growth of cloned, 100, 102
optimal ratio of fragment to vector, 111
purification, from agarose gels, 207–209
reamplification of, 109–110
separation of amplified, 100, 101, 102
size and migration rate, 206
subcloning, 196–204

DNA inserts, 112, 152, 153, 196–200

DNA libraries, commercial, 140. *See also* Library screening

DNA polymerase, 2. *See also Taq* DNA polymerase
basic considerations, 28–30
handling reagent, 8–9

DNA primers. *See* Primers

DNA probes, 89, 139, 165

DNA-protein interactions
altered gene expression with DD-PCR, 113–117
electrophoresis and, 148–149
selection and binding sites technique, 145–152

DNase I, 103, 104, 117

DNA sequence, 9–21, 218

DNASTAR, 215, 217

DNA template, 2–3, 5–6

dNTP. *See* Deoxyribonucleotide triphosphate

Dot-blot analysis, 43, 89, 100–101, 113–117

Downstream primer, definition, 44

Duplex, 21–22, 33

Dupont NEN, 217

Dyes. *See* Stains and dyes

E

Economic factors, of primer synthesis, 28
EcoRV restriction enzyme sites, 123
EDTA
 in direct sequencing by PCR, 155, 157, 158
 in dot-blot differential hybridization, 117
 in electrophoresis of DNA-protein complex, 149
 in elution from wells of agarose gel, 209
 in extraction of genomic DNA, 181, 182
 in isolation of plasmid DNA, 185
 in isolation of total RNA, 189, 190
 in multiplex PCR for genotyping, 174
 in preparation of insert DNA, 199
 in purification of mRNA, 193, 194
 in reporter gene analysis, 94, 95
Electronic files
 digitized images, 68
 editing and storage of, 16, 19–21
 on GenBank, 16, 19, 21
 for PRIMER software, 26
Electronic subtraction (ES), 100
Electrophoresis, of DNA, 205–209
Electrophoretic mobility shift assays (EMSA), 146, 159
Electroporation, 209
ELISA, 166
Elongation, 30
Elongation temperature
 basic cloning by RT-PCR, 129
 construction of wild-type plasmid, 56
 cycle-based quantitative RT-PCR, 81
 direct sequencing by PCR, 156
 generation of wild-type plasmid, 58, 59
 hot start, 62, 68, 73
 internal standard amplification, 46, 50, 52
 library screening, 141, 143, 145
 multiplex PCR for genotyping, 174
 NAT2 genotyping, 170
 PCR amplification, 106
 PCR clone check, 154
 RACE, 136, 137, 139
 selection and binding sites technique, 150, 151

semiquantitative RT-PCR, 85
 standard RT-PCR, 62
Elution, from wells of agarose gels, 208–209
EMSA (electrophoretic mobility shift assays), 146, 159
"End cutter," 127, 147
Endonuclease, restriction, 53, 127
Enrichment screening, 142–144
Enzymes, storage of, 8–9
Enzyme sites, mutated restriction, 52–59. *See also* Restriction enzymes
Epitopes, 126
Eppendorf, 217
Equipment, separation of pre-PCR and post-PCR, 7
Equivalency point. *See* Crossover point
Ericomp, 213
ES. *See* External standard
Escherichia coli
 DH5α cells, 57, 125, 131, 201, 202
 in differential display PCR, 102
 heat-shock transformation of, 57, 111, 125, 131, 201
 JM109 cells, 201
 size of genome and copies per microgram, 31
ES (electronic subtraction), 100
Ethidium bromide stain
 advantages/disadvantages, 207
 of cDNA fragments, 110
 in elution from wells of agarose gel, 209
 in ligation, 200
 overall strategy, 31, 64
 in PCR protocol, 174, 175
 of rRNA, 104
 warning, 206
EuGene Primer Design Software, 217
European Molecular Biology Laboratory, 10
Exons
 in amplification across an intron, 50
 in reporter gene analysis, 94
Exonuclease activity, 3′ to 5,′ 123
Exponential phase, 5
Extension, 29–30. *See also* Elongation temperature
External standard (ES)
 in cycle-based quantitative RT-PCR, 76

Index

definition, 44
selection of, 82
External standard RT-PCR
(semiquantitative), 82–85, 92

F

False priming sites, on OLIGO software,
24–25
Fast green stain, 88
Ficoll loading buffer, 96, 116, 160, 209
Fidelity, basic considerations, 29
Filters
nylon, 82, 113
Whatman DE81, 78
Whatman 3MM, 106, 117, 149
Fingerprinting, RNA, 100, 107
First-strand buffer, 108, 117
Fisher Biotech, 86
Fisher Scientific, 214, 217
FITC-conjugated primers, 107
5′-terminus of the oligonucleotide, 3
amplification of, 134, 137–139, 144
sequences added onto, 45, 122
Fluorescence image analyzer, 107
FMC Bioproducts, 214, 217
FMC Corporation, 109
Formaldehyde agarose gel, 104
Formamide, 26, 37, 106, 160, 181–182
Formamide loading buffer, 115
Forward exchange buffer, 95, 157
Forward primer (FP)
in basic cloning by RT-PCR, 126–127,
128
BG, 172, 173
in competitive quantitative RT-PCR
procedure, 67, 72
in construction of wild-type plasmid,
55
in cycle-based quantitative RT-PCR, 80
definition, 44
in dot-blot differential hybridization,
116
5′ labeling of, 77–78
gene-specific, in RACE, 136
GSTM1, 172, 173
GSTT1, 172, 173
in internal standard amplification, 49,
51
in library screening, 140, 141, 143

in NAT2 genotyping, 167, 168, 169
oligonucleotides in SAAB, 147
in PCR clone check, 153
plasmid-specific, 53, 58, 59, 152, 153
in quantitation of hnRNA, 90
in recombinant RNA synthesis, 45, 46
in reporter gene analysis, 93, 94
in semiquantitative RT-PCR, 84
in *in situ* RT-PCR, 87
in standard RT-PCR, 61
FP. *See* Forward primer
Freeze-and-squeeze method, 207–208

G

Galactose, 205
β-Galactosidase, 91, 93, 203
GAPDH (glyceraldehyde phosphate
dehydrogenase), 44, 82
GC content
on OLIGO software, 23, 24
target characteristics and, 21
Gel casting tray, 208
Gel combs, 208
Gel electrophoresis, separation of
amplified DNA fragments in, 100,
101, 102
Gelman Sciences, Inc., 217
Gel shift assay, 148, 150, 151
Gel shift buffer, 148, 158
GenBank, 9, 102
access through Internet Email, 10–16
access through World Wide Web sites,
16–21
GeneAmp PCR System, 170, 174
General Biotechnology indexes, 218
General competitive RT-PCR, 64–69, 90
Gene-specific primer 3 (GSP3), 51
Gene-specific primer 5 (GSP5), 51
Gene-specific primers (GSP)
in construction of an internal standard
using mutagenesis, 53
in library screening, 141, 143, 144
in RACE, 134, 136, 137, 138
GenHunter, 103, 105. *See also* DNase I
Genomes, sizes of, 31
Genomic analysis
of carcinogen metabolism
polymorphisms, 164–165
high-throughput, 165–167

Genomic DNA
  extraction by formamide, 181–182
  extraction with solvents, 179–181
Genosys Biotechnologies, Inc., 105, 109, 214, 217
Genotype analysis, 163–175
Gibco-BRL, 114, 125, 128, 202
Glassware, 7–8
Glass wool, 47, 50, 56, 58
β-Globin, 94, 165, 167, 172
Glogos II, 107
Gloves, 7, 8
Glucose, 182, 185
Glutathione S-transferase (GST), 164, 165
Glutathione S-transferase M1 (GSTM1), 167, 172–175
Glutathione S-transferase T1 (GSTT1), 167, 172–175
Glyceraldehyde phosphate dehydrogenase (GAPDH), 44, 82
Glycerol
  in bacterial transformation, 201
  in direct sequencing by PCR, 159
  in dot-blot differential hybridization, 115, 116
  in electrophoresis of DNA-protein complexes, 149
  enchancement of PCR by, 37
  enzyme storage in, 8
  in purification of DNA fragments, 209
Glycerol loading buffer, 209
Glycerol shock solution, 210, 211
Glycogen, 149
GSP. *See* Gene-specific primers
GST. *See* Glutathione S-transferase
Guanidium thiocyanate, 186–187, 189–190, 192

H

Hairpin loops, 25
Heated-lid thermocyclers, 30
Heat shock
  in cloning amplified fragments, 111
  in control ligation reaction, 57, 125, 131
  preparation of competent cells for, 201
  protocols, 201–202
HEPES buffered saline (HBS), 210, 211

HEPES-KOH, 95, 157
Heterogeneous nuclear RNA (hnRNA), 89–90
High-throughput genotyping, 165–167
Hipopurine ribose transferase (HPRT), 82
Historical background, 2–3
Hitachi Software, 217
hnRNA (heterogeneous nuclear RNA), 89–90
Hoods, 7
Hot start PCR, 10, 34
  in NAT2 genotyping, 170
  optimization experiment, 33–35
  protocol, 34, 62, 67–68, 72–73, 80–81, 84–85, 129
HotStart technique, by Perkin-Elmer, 33
Housekeeping genes, 82
HPRT (hipopurine ribose transferase), 82
Human genome, 31, 164
Hybaid, 217, 218
Hybond-N+ nylon membrane, 113
Hybridization sites, 45

I

Identi-kit, 107
Inosine-containing primers, 132–133
Insert DNA. *See* DNA inserts
Insert-specific primers, 152, 153
In situ RT-PCR, 86–88
Internal standard (IS)
  amplification efficiency of, *vs.* target, 63, 77
  amplification of, 46–47, 77
    across an intron, 50–52
    low-stringency, 48–50
  avoidance of contamination by, 60, 65, 70, 79
  construction, 44–63
    with a mutated restriction enzyme site, 52–59
    recombinant RNA synthesis, 45–48
    testing, 60–63
  definition, 43
  in reporter gene analysis, 94
  role in competitive quantitative RT-PCR, 64, 65
  role in competitive RT-PCR using a standard curve, 69, 73–76

Index

227

International Nucleotide Sequence
Database Collaboration, 10
International Union of Biochemistry
(IUB), 132, 133
Internet addresses
browser software, 16
companies, catalogs and resources, 10,
217–218
GenBank, 10, 16–21
PRIMER software, 26, 28
Intra-strand complementarity, 21
Introns
amplification across, 50–52
in heterogeneous RNA, 89, 90
in reporter gene analysis, 94
Invitrogen Corporation, 110, 213, 218
In vitro transcription, 52, 59
protocol, 47–48
rabbit reticulocyte lysate and, 146
IPTG, 126, 131, 158, 202, 204
IS. *See* Internal standard
Isoamyl alcohol, 149, 184, 185, 186, 187,
193, 199
Isolation and purification
of genomic DNA from animals,
179–182
of plasmid DNA, 182–186
of RNA, 186–196
suppliers, 214–215

J

JM109 cells, 201

K

Kanamycin, 111
Kinetic approach (cycle-based
quantitative RT-PCR), 76–82
Klenow DNA polymerase, 147
Klenow fragment, 147
Klenow 10X buffer, 147
Kpn I, 171, 175

L

Labeling. *See* Radiolabeling
Laboratory considerations, 6–9, 165,
166
lacZ gene, 111, 197, 203

Lambda control polymerase chain
reaction, 4
Lambda phage arms, 140
Laminar flow hoods, 7
Layout of laboratory, 6–7
LB buffer. *See* Luria-Bertaini
buffer/medium
LB plates, 158, 183
Liang and Pardee method, 100, 103–107
Library RACE, 144–145
Library screening, 100, 101, 122
Life Technologies, 218
Ligase buffer, 95, 157, 200
Ligation
of cDNA fragments, 111–112
of PCR product, 125–126
of plasmid vector and insert DNA,
199–200
Ligation buffer, 56, 57, 111, 115, 125, 131
Ligation reaction
in bacterial transformation, 201
in basic cloning by RT-PCR, 130–131
components of, 200
in construction of wild-type plasmid,
56–57
self-ligated vector, 125
Linear regression
absorbance unit ratio *vs.* concentration
ratio, 75
quantitation of target mRNA and
internal standard, 69, 74
Linker gene
alternative to using, 48–50
definition, 44
in recombinant RNA synthesis, 45
Lithium chloride, 188–189, 193, 194
Loading dye, 81, 141, 143, 145, 154, 171,
175, 206
Low abundance messages. *See* Rare
messages
Low-stringency amplification, 48–50
Luciferase, 91, 93, 94
Luria-Bertaini buffer/medium (LB)
in bacterial transformation, 200, 201,
202, 204–205
in direct sequencing by PCR, 158
in isolation of plasmid DNA, 183, 184,
185
in library screening by PCR, 142
Lysis buffer, 181–182, 185

M

Magnesium chloride
  in basic cloning by RT-PCR, 127, 128
  in cDNA synthesis, 87, 108
  in competitive quantitative RT-PCR procedure, 65, 66, 67
  in competitive RT-PCR with standard curve, 70, 71, 72
  in construction of a PCR cloning vector, 54
  in construction of TA cloning vector, 124
  in construction of wild-type plasmid, 55
  in cycle-based quantitative RT-PCR, 79, 80
  in digestion of contaminating cDNA in RNA, 104
  in dot-blot differential hybridization, 115, 116
  in hot start procotol, 34
  in internal standard amplification, 46, 49, 51
  in library screening, 140, 143, 144
  in magnesium ion concentration optimization experiment, 35–36
  in multiplex PCR for genotyping, 173, 175
  in NAT2 genotyping, 169
  in oil-overlay thermocycler protocol, 30
  in PCR clone check, 153
  in PCR mutagenesis, 57, 59
  in preparation of insert DNA, 199
  in RACE, 135, 137
  in reporter gene analysis, 92, 93, 95
  in selection and binding sites technique, 150, 151
  selection of transformants and, 204
  in semiquantitative RT-PCR, 83, 84
  in *in situ* RT-PCR, 87, 88
  in Sokolov and Prockop method, 108
  in standard RT-PCR procedure, 60, 61
Magnesium ion concentration, 2
  dNTP and, 29, 30, 37
  optimization experiment, 35–36
Magnesium sulfate, 158, 201, 202, 203
Maltose, 201

Manganese ion, 2
Marker gene, 197
Mathematical considerations, 3–5
β-Mercaptoethanol, 94, 111, 155, 174, 186, 192
Messenger RNA. *See* mRNA
Metaphor, 109
Methods. *See* Protocols
MicroAmp, 112
MicroAmp Reaction Tray, 174
MicroAmp Reaction Tubes, 174
Migration rate, 206
Millipore Corporation, 215, 218
Mineral oil, 38, 86–87, 106, 117
MJ Research, Inc., 213
MMLV reverse transcriptase buffer, 61, 95
  in basic cloning by RT-PCR, 128
  in competitive quantitative RT-PCR procedure, 66
  in competitive RT-PCR with standard curve, 71
  in direct sequencing by PCR, 157
  in dot-blot differential hybridization, 115
  in RACE, 135, 137
  in reporter gene analysis, 92
  in reverse transcription, 105
  in semiquantitative RT-PCR, 83
  in *in situ* RT-PCR, 87
Moloney murine leukemia virus reverse transcriptase (MoMuLV), 117
Monoclonal antibodies, 33
Mouse, size of genome and copies per microgram, 31
M13(-20) plasmid, 144
M13(rev) plasmid, 144
MRC Corporation, 107
mRNA (messenger RNA)
  in cDNA synthesis, 108
  differential expression of. *See* Differential display PCR
  levels of, *vs.* transcription rate, 89
  purification of, by oligo(dT)-cellulose column, 190–195
  quantitation, 43
  of reporter gene, 91, 93–96
MRRP (mutant reverse primers), 53–54
Msp I, 171, 175

Index

Mullis, Kary, 2, 3
Multiplex PCR, 165–166, 167, 172–175
Mutagenesis
  contruction of an internal standard
    using, 52–59
  role of, in known binding site, 146
  in RT-PCR, multiple samples *vs.* high
    cycle number, 127
Mutant reverse primer (MRRP), 53–54
Mutated restriction enzyme sites, 52–59

N

National Biosciences, Inc., 22, 23–26
National Center for Biotechnology
    Information (NCBI), 10, 218. *See*
    also Genbank
National Instruments, 218
NAT (N-acetyltransferase), 164
NAT2 (N-acetyltransferase 2), 164,
    167–172, 175
NCBI (National Center for Biotechnology
    Information), 10, 218
Nested primer design, 89, 90, 126, 144
Netscape, 10
Neutralizing solution, 117
New England Biolabs, Inc., 213, 218
Nitrocellulose membranes, 139
Nontarget products, 33
Northern blot analysis, 43, 100, 115, 186
Not1 restriction endonuclease site, 127
Novagen, Inc., 213, 218
Nuclear run-on assay, 89
Nucleotides, choice of, 104–105, 132
Nylon membrane, 82, 113

O

Oil-overlay thermocyclers, basic
    protocol, 30–31
OLA (oligo-ligation assay), 166–167
Oligo(dT)12-18 primer, 114
Oligo(dT)15 primer, 61
  in basic cloning by RT-PCR, 128
  in competitive quantitative RT-PCR
    procedure, 66
  in competitive RT-PCR with standard
    curve, 70, 71
  in cycle-based quantitative RT-PCR, 79
  in reporter gene analysis, 92

in semiquantitative RT-PCR, 83
  in *in situ* RT-PCR, 87
Oligo(dT)17-adapter primer, in RACE,
    135, 138
Oligo(dT) primers
  anchored, 100, 104, 105, 106, 117
  in cellulose column, purification of
    mRNA with, 190–195
  in RACE, 134, 135
Oligo-ligation assay (OLA), 166–167
Oligonucleotide primers. *See* Primers
Oligonucleotides
  in selection and binding sites
    technique, 147–148, 150, 151
  suppliers, 214
  synthesis of, 28
OLIGO software, 22, 23–26
Online resources, 217–218. *See also*
    Internet addresses
Operon Technologies, Inc., 105, 214, 218
Optimization experiments
  additives and other approaches, 37–38
  annealing temperature, 32–33
  cycle number, 31–32
  DNA sample for, 31
  hot start, 33–35
  magnesium chloride concentration,
    35–36
Overhang vectors, 122, 123

P

Paraffin, 86
PBS. *See* Phosphate-buffered saline
PCR. *See* Polymerase chain reaction
PCR Applications Manual, 218
PCR buffer II, 37
PCR cloning, 54–55
PCRII vector, 110, 111, 112
PCR Primers Database Home Page,
    218
PCR product
  amount, calculation of, 55, 76, 125, 130
  cloning, 50, 53
  cloning vector, construction of, 54–55
  with different secondary structure,
    comparison of, 76
  of different size than target DNA,
    48–50
  extraneous, 33

ligation of, 125–126, 131
on OLIGO software, 23, 24
Pedro's BioMolecular Research Tools, 218
PEG, 37
Perfect Match, 37
Perkin-Elmer Corporation, The, 33, 106, 112, 213, 218
Pfu, 21, 29
Phage, library screening with, 139–140
Phage plaques, 139, 142, 144
Phage-specific primer, 144
Pharmacia Biotech, 112, 214, 218
Phenol
  in genomic DNA extraction from tissue, 180
  in purification of mRNA, 193
  in rapid isolation of total RNA, 187
  warnings, 187, 193
Phenol/chloroform buffer
  in direct sequencing by PCR, 158
  in dot-blot differential hybridization, 117
  in extraction of DNA, 204
  LiCl-urea and phenol-chloroform RNA extraction, 188–189
  in ligation reaction, 130
  in preparation of insert DNA, 199
  in preparation of plasmid DNA, 184, 186
  in reporter gene analysis, 96
Phenol/chloroform/isoamyl alcohol, 149, 189
Phosphate-buffered saline (PBS)
  in genomic DNA extraction, 179, 180, 182
  in transfection, 210, 211
Photography, 68, 93, 110, 200, 203, 207
Physical hot start, 33, 34
Pipettes, 7–8
Pipetting techniques, 9
  dot-blot analysis, 113
  library screening, 141
  robotic, 167
Pipettors, calibration of, 9
Plasmid/phage-specific primer, 144
Plasmids
  in construction of a PCR cloning vector, 54–55

in construction of T-overhand vector, 123–124
isolation and purification of DNA, 182–186
ligation of plasmid vector, 199–200
PCR clone check and, 152–154
recombinant, selection of transformants containing, 202–204
in reporter gene analysis, 91, 93–96
wild-type, 53, 55–57, 58, 59
Plasmid-specific forward primer (PSPFP), 53, 58, 59
Plasmid-specific primers, 152, 153
Plasmid vector, ligation of, 199–200
Plasticware, 8
Plateau phase, 5–6, 31
Plotting
  absorbance unit ratio, 75
  5′ labeling of PCR primer, 82
  quantitation of target mRNA *vs.* internal standard, 68–69, 74
  yield *vs.* cycle number, 77
Polyacrylamide gel, samples cut from, 100
Polyadenylation signals, 126
Polyadenylation site, 89
Poly(A) RNA, 117
  extraction, 107
  in RACE, 134
  preparation of, 103–104
  sites, 51
Poly(A)+ RNA, 127
  amount, calculation of, 196
  purification of, 190–195
Poly(A)+ tails, 45
PolyATract mRNA Isolation System, 107
Poly(dI-dC)-poly(dI-dC), 159
Polymerase. *See* DNA polymerase; *Taq* DNA polymerase
Polymerase chain reaction laboratory, 6–9, 165, 166
Polymerase chain reaction (PCR). *See also* PCR product; Reverse transcription polymerase chain reaction
  allele-specific, 164–165, 166
  anchored, 122. *See also* Oligo(dT) primers, anchored

Index

231

basic considerations, 28–30
buffers. *See* Buffers
clone check, 152–154
cloning by, 121–160
colony, 112
degenerate primer, 131–134
differential display, 99–117
direct sequencing by, 154–160
historical background, 2–3
mathematical considerations, 3–5
multiplex, 165–166, 167, 172–175
mutagenesis, 57–59
with RFLP, 164–165, 167–172
theory, 3–6
Polymorphisms
analysis using PCR, 167–175
of carcinogen metabolism, 164
PolyT, in RACE, 134
Poly T tail, 53, 55
Polyvinylpyrrolidone, 116
Population-based studies, 165
Potassium acetate, 184, 185
Potassium chloride
in digestion of contaminating cDNA,
104
in direct sequencing by PCR, 155, 157
in DNA extraction, 182
in dot-blot differential hybridization,
115, 116
in reporter gene analysis, 95
in transfection of mammalian cells, 211
PPARα gene, 64
Prehybridization solutions, 114, 116
Premier Biosoft International, 215
Prime-It II random primer labeling kit,
114
Primer dimers, formation, 22
Primers, 2–3. *See also* Forward primer;
Reverse primer
allele specific, 164–165
characteristics, 21–22
choice of, in reverse transcription,
104–105
degenerate, 131–134
design of, 21–28
with OLIGO software, 23–26
with PRIMER software, 26–28
evaluation of peptide sequences for,
132

FITC-conjugated, 107
5′ labeling of, 77–78
inosine-containing, 132–133
insert-specific, 152, 153
internal *vs.* 3′ terminal stability for, 25
mutagenic, 58
nested, 89, 90, 126, 144
oligo(dT) primers, anchored, 100, 104,
105, 106, 117
plasmid-specific, 53, 58, 59, 152, 153
radioactive, 63, 76, 77–78
RTase, 89, 90
in Sokolov and Prockop method, 109
suppliers, 215
synthesis, 28
PRIMER software, 22, 26–28, 29
Priming efficiency, on OLIGO software,
24–25
Probe, DNA, 89, 139, 165
Probe-On slides, 86
Promega Corporation
address, 214
DNase I, 103, 104, 117
glass wool, 47, 50, 56, 58
PolyATract mRNA Isolation System,
107
Taq DNA polymerase, sequencing
grade, 155
TnT kit, 146
"Proof-reading," 123
Proteinase K, 180, 194
Protein-DNA interactions. *See* Selection
and binding sites technique
Protocols
amplification
of cDNA 3′ ends, 135–137
of cDNA 5′ ends, 137–139
of a dilution series of rcRNA,
60–63
of internal standard, 46–47, 49–50
PCR, 106–107, 169–170
bacterial transformations, 200–204
cloning
of amplified cDNA fragments,
110–112
construction of PCR cloning vector,
54–55
construction of TA cloning vector,
123–126

PCR clone check, 152–154
  by RT-PCR, 127–131
colony-PCR, 112
constant RNA with serial dilutions of
  internal standard, 65–68
degenerate primer PCR, 133–134
detection of reporter plasmid DNA in
  reporter gene analysis, 93–96
digestion of contaminating cDNA in
  RNA, 104
direct sequencing by PCR, 154–160
electrophoresis
  agarose gel, 206–209
  of DNA, 206–209
elution from wells of agarose gels,
  208–209
extraction of DNA, 179–182, 204
hnRNA, quantitation of, 89–90
insert DNA, preparation of, 198–199
library screening
  dilution screening, 140–142
  enrichment screening, 142–144
  library RACE, 144–145
luciferase levels in reporter gene
  analysis, 91–93
NAT2 genotyping, 169–171
oil-overlay thermocyclers, 30–31
PCR mutagenesis, 57–59
plasmid DNA, preparation of,
  183–186
purification
  of DNA fragments from agarose
    gels, 207–209
  of poly(A)+RNA from total RNA,
    190–195
rapid isolation of total RNA, 186–190
restriction digest, 170–171
reverse transcription, 105
RNA, measurement of, 195–196
RT-PCR
  competitive, with standard curve,
    70–73
  cycle-based quantitative, 77–82
  semiquantitative, 83–85
  in situ, 86–88
selection and binding sites technique,
  147–152
selection of transformants containing
  recombinant plasmids,
  202–204

transcription, in vitro, 47–48
transfection of mammal cells, 209–211
transformation, 201–202
vectors, preparation of, 197–198
wild-type plasmid, generation of,
  55–57
PSPFP (plasmid-specific forward primer),
  53, 58, 59
Purification. See Isolation and purification

Q

Quantitation detection, calculations and
    plotting
  cycle-based quantitative RT-PCR,
    81–82
  general competitive RT-PCR, 68–69
  semiquantitative RT-PCR, 85
  using a standard curve, 73–76
Quantitative RT-PCR
  competitive, 63–76
  cycle-based, 76–82

R

Rabbit reticulocyte lysate, 146
RACE (rapid amplification of cDNA
    ends), 101, 122, 134–139,
    144–145
Radioactive primers, 63, 76, 77–78
Radioactive probes, 89, 139, 165
Radiolabeling
  autoradiography, 82, 107
  in differential display PCR, 100
  DNA probes, 89, 139, 165
  of nucleic acid, 89
  of primers, 63, 76, 77–78
Ransom Hill Bioscience, Inc., 214,
    218
Rapid amplification of cDNA ends
    (RACE), 101, 122, 134–139,
    144–145
Rare messages, 103
rcRNA (recombinant RNA)
  amplification of a dilution series of,
    60–63
  handling, 60, 65, 70, 79
  synthesis, construction of internal
    standard, 45–48
Reagents. See also Buffers

Index

233

contamination of, 6, 7
handling of, 8–9
Reamplification, of cDNA fragment,
  109–110
Recombinant RNA. *See* rcRNA
Reference genes, 82
Reporter gene, analysis, 91–96
Reporter gene expression, 43
Research Genetics, 214, 218
Resources, 213–215
Restriction enzyme buffer, 123, 130, 154
Restriction enzymes
  in basic cloning by RT-PCR, 127, 130
  in construction of internal standard, 53
  digestion of vector and DNA insert for
    subcloning, 196–199
  digestion protocol, 170–171
  double-digestion reaction, 197
  in library screening, 139
  in NAT2 genotyping, 170–171
  suppliers, 213
Restriction enzyme sites
  in choosing a TA cloning vector, 123
  in cloning by RT-PCR, 126
  mutated, 52–59
  in NAT2 genotyping, 168
  polymorphisms at, 164
Restriction fragment length
    polymorphism (RFLP), 164
Reticulocyte lysate, 146
Reverse primer (RP)
  in basic cloning by RT-PCR, 126–127,
    128
  BG, 172, 173
  in competitive quantitative RT-PCR
    procedure, 67
  in competitive RT-PCR with standard
    curve, 72
  in construction of wild-type plasmid,
    55
  in cycle-based quantitative RT-PCR, 80
  definition, 44
  in dot-blot differential hybridization,
    116
  5' labeling of, 77–78
  gene-specific, in RACE, 137, 138
  GSTM1, 172, 173
  GSTT1, 172, 173
  in internal standard amplification, 49,
    51

in library screening, 140, 141, 143
mutant reverse, 53–54
in NAT2 genotyping, 167, 168, 169
oligonucleotides in SAAB, 147
in PCR clone check, 153
in quantitation of hnRNA, 90
in recombinant RNA synthesis, 45, 46
in reporter gene analysis, 93, 94
in semiquantitative RT-PCR, 84
in *in situ* RT-PCR, 87
in standard RT-PCR procedure, 61
Reverse transcriptase. *See also* AMV
    reverse transcriptase; MMLV
    reverse transcriptase buffer
  handling reagent, 8–9
  Moloney murine leukemia virus, 117
  SuperScript II, 114, 128
  suppliers, 213
Reverse transcription
  in Liang and Pardee method, 104–105
  in RACE, 137
Reverse transcription polymerase chain
    reaction (RT-PCR)
  basic cloning by, 126–131
  quantitative, 43
    competitive, 63–76
    cycle-based, 76–82
    semiquantitative, 82–85
    in situ, 43, 86–88
    standard procedures, 60–63
RFLP (restriction fragment length
    polymorphism), 164
Ribosomal RNA, 104
RNA. *See also* mRNA; Poly(A)+ RNA;
    Poly(A) RNA; rcRNA; Total RNA
  extraction solution, 193
  heterogeneous nuclear, 89–90
  internal standard with poly(A)+ tail, 45
  isolation and purification of, 186–196
  measurement of, 195–196
  ribosomal, 104
  storage of, 8–9
RNA buffer, 193
RNA fingerprinting, 100, 107
RNA polymerase
  T7 RNA polymerase sites, 50, 51, 115
  in *in vitro* transcription, 47
RNA polymerase sites, 45
RNase, 103, 182, 183, 184, 186
RNase inhibitor, 8–9, 104, 117

234 PCR Protocols in Molecular Toxicology

RNase protection assays, 43
RNA synthesis. *See* rcRNA, synthesis
RP. *See* Reverse primer
rRNA (ribosomal RNA), 104
rRNasin, 61
  in basic cloning by RT-PCR, 128
  in cDNA synthesis, 108
  in competitive quantitative RT-PCR
    procedure, 66
  in competitive RT-PCR with standard
    curve, 71
  in cycle-based quantitative RT-PCR, 79
  in RACE, 135, 137
  in reporter gene analysis, 92
  in semiquantitative RT-PCR, 83
  in *in situ* RT-PCR, 87
RTase primer, 89, 90
RT-PCR. *See* Reverse transcription
    polymerase chain reaction
Rx buffers, 30, 34, 36, 37, 46

S

SAAB (selection and binding sites
    technique), 145–152
SAGE (serial analysis of gene
    expression), 100
Salmon sperm, 116
Sarcosyl, 192
SDS. *See* Sodium dodecyl sulfate
Search strategy
  Genbank through Email access,
    11–15
  Genbank through World Wide Web
    sites, 16–19, 20
  for primers on PRIMER software,
    26–28
Secondary structure, comparison of
    products with different, 76
Selection and binding sites technique
    (SAAB), 145–152
Semiquantitative RT-PCR, 82–85, 92
Sequencing buffer, 159
Serial analysis of gene expression
    (SAGE), 100
"Short" product, formula, 4
SH (subtractive hybridization), 100, 102,
    103
Sigma Chemical Company, 214, 218
Signal detection, 88

Silica chips, 165
Silver stain, 107
Single nucleotide polymorphisms (SNP),
    164
Slides
  preparation for *in situ* RT-PCR, 86
  Probe-On, 86
Slot-blot analysis, 43, 89, 100, 115
SmaI restriction enzyme site, 123
SM buffer, 142, 144, 158
SNP (single nucleotide polymorphisms),
    164
Sodium acetate, 204
Sodium acetate buffer, 117, 189, 190,
    192–193, 199
Sodium citrate, 116, 182, 192
Sodium dodecyl sulfate (SDS), 182, 185,
    188, 189, 193, 194
Sodium lauryl sarcosinate, 189
Software
  EuGene Primer Design, 217
  Hitachi, 217
  OLIGO, 22, 23–26
  PRIMER, 22, 26–28, 29
  primer selection, 22–28
  World Wide Web browser, 16
Sokolov and Prockop method, 101–102,
    107–109
Southern blot analysis, 126, 164
Specificity, basic considerations, 29
Spermidine, 37, 95, 157, 199
SP6 plasmid, 144, 153, 196
SSC, 113, 114, 116
Stability of a primer, internal *vs.* 3'
    terminal, 25
Stains and dyes. *See also* Ethidium
    bromide stain; Loading dye;
    Xylene cyanol
  bromophenol blue, 96, 115, 159, 160,
    209
  cresol red, 116
  fast green, 88
  for signal detection, 88
  silver, 107
Standard competitive RT-PCR, 64–69, 90
"Standard PCR," protocol, 34
Sterilization of glassware, 8
Stock reagents. *See* Buffers; Reagents
Stop solution, 160
Storage, rcRNA, 60, 65, 70, 79

Index   **235**

Storage temperature
  in basic cloning by RT-PCR, 129
  in construction of wild-type plasmid,
    56
  in cycle-based quantitative RT-PCR, 81
  in direct sequencing by PCR, 156
  in generation of wild-type plasmid, 58,
    59
  in hot start, 62, 68, 73
  in internal standard amplification, 50,
    52
  in library screening, 141, 143, 145
  in PCR amplification, 106
  in PCR clone check, 154
  in RACE, 137, 139
  in selection and binding sites
    technique, 150, 151
  in semiquantitative RT-PCR, 85
  in standard RT-PCR, 62
Stratagene, 32, 37, 107, 114
StrataLinker, 114
Subcloning, 45, 196–204
  digestion of vector and DNA insert for,
    196–199
  DNA sequences added onto 5′-
    terminus, 122
Subtractive hybridization (SH), 100, 102,
  103
SuperScript II reverse transcriptase, 114,
  128
Suppliers, 213–215

T

TA cloning, 53, 122–126, 145
TA Cloning kit, 110, 111
TAE buffer, 206, 207, 208
Tailing buffer, 138
Taq DNA polymerase, 37
  activity at low temperatures, 33
  in basic cloning by RT-PCR, 129, 130
  in cold start, 68, 73, 85, 130
  in competitive quantitative RT-PCR,
    67, 68
  in competitive RT-PCR with standard
    curve, 72, 73
  in construction of a PCR cloning
    vector, 55
  in construction of TA cloning vector,
    124

  in construction of wild-type plasmid,
    56
  in cycle-based quantitative RT-PCR,
    80, 81
  denaturation of, 21
  in dot-blot differential hybridization,
    117
  in generation of wild-type plasmid, 58
  in hot start, 34, 62, 67, 72, 80, 81, 85,
    129
  in internal standard amplification, 46,
    49, 52
  in library screening, 141, 143, 145
  in magnesium ion concentration
    optimization experiment, 36
  in multiplex PCR for genotyping, 173,
    175
  in NAT2 genotyping, 169
  in oil-overlay thermocycler protocol,
    31
  in PCR amplification, Liang and Pardee
    method, 106
  in PCR clone check, 153
  in RACE, 136, 139
  in reamplification of cDNA fragments,
    110
  in reporter gene analysis, 93
  in selection and binding sites
    technique, 150, 151
  in semiquantitative RT-PCR, 85
  sequencing grade, in direct sequencing
    by PCR, 155
  in *in situ* RT-PCR, 88
  in Sokolov and Prockop method,
    109
  in standard RT-PCR procedure, 62, 63
  suppliers, 213
Taq I, 171, 175
TaqStart antibody, 33, 34, 35, 36, 38, 174
TaqStart buffer, 35
Target gene
  definition, 44
  determination in dilution series, 65
  expression of, relative to housekeeping
    gene, 82
Target mRNA
  in amplification across an intron, 51
  calculation, using standard curve,
    73–76
  plotting, 69

236 PCR Protocols in Molecular Toxicology

Target region
  characteristics, 21
  on PRIMER software, 26
TBE buffer, 149, 206, 207, 208
TBS buffer, 86, 88
TBS-MS buffer, 88
TE buffer
  in cycle-based quantitative RT-PCR, 78
  in direct sequencing by PCR, 157
  in extraction of genomic DNA, 179, 180
  in isolation of total RNA, 190
  in measurement of RNA, 195
  in preparation of insert DNA, 199
  in preparation of plasmid DNA, 184, 185
  in purification of poly(A)+RNA, 194
  in reporter gene analysis, 95
  in selection of transformants, 204
TEMED, 149
Template, definition, 44
Terminal d transferase, 138
T4 DNA ligase, 57, 111, 125, 131, 200
T4 polynucleotide kinase, 78, 148
T4 polynucleotide kinase buffer, 148, 157
Theory, 3–6
Thermocycle programs
  amplification across an intron, 52
  amplification of dilution series rcRNA, 61
  basic cloning by RT-PCR, 128
  cDNA synthesis, 108
  colony-PCR, 112
  competitive RT-PCR, 66, 71
  cycle-based quantitative RT-PCR, 79
  direct sequencing by PCR, 156
  DNA sample for optimization, 32–33, 35, 36
  generation of wild-type plasmid, 56
  hot start, 62, 68, 73, 81, 85
  internal standard amplification, 46, 49–50
  library screening, 141, 143, 145
  multiplex PCR for genotyping, 174
  NAT2 genotyping, 170
  PCR amplification, 106, 109
  PCR clone check, 153–154
  PCR mutagenesis, 58, 59
  RACE, 136–137, 139
  reporter gene analysis, 92

selection and binding sites technique, 150, 151
semi-quantitative RT-PCR, 83
signal detection, 88
Thermocyclers
  heated-lid, 30
  interruption of, during cycle-based quantitative RT-PCR, 76, 79, 81
  oil-overlay, 30–31
  parameter settings for, 35, 36
  Perkin-Elmer 9600, 106, 112, 170, 174
  Strategene, 32
  suppliers, 213
  as surrogate heat block, 62, 72, 80, 85
3'-terminus of the oligonucleotide, 2
  in allele-specific PCR, 164–165
  amplification of, 134, 135–137, 144
  complementary regions at, and target region selection, 22
  terminal vs. internal stability, 25
Tissue
  culture plates for isolation of RNA, 91
  extraction of genomic DNA from, 180–181
  LiCl-urea and phenol-chloroform RNA extraction from, 188
  rapid isolation of total RNA from, 187
Tissue distribution, 43
TnT kit, 146
Total RNA, 105, 127
  amount, calculation of, 196
  in basic cloning by RT-PCR, 128
  isolation with guanidium thiocyanate, 189–190
  preparation of, 103–104
  purification of poly(A)+RNA from, 190–195
  rapid isolation of, 186–190
T-overhang vectors, 122, 123
T7 plasmid, 144
Transcription. See also In vitro transcription
  activation, 43
  inhibitor, 90
  rate of, 89–90
Transcription buffer, 95, 157
Transfection, of mammal cells, 209–211
Transformation. See also Heat shock
  bacterial, 200–201
  calcium chloride, 201, 202

Index

selection of transformants containing recombinant plasmids, 202–204
using calcium chloride method, 202
using heat shock method, 201–202
Translation stop and start sites, 126
TriReagent, 107
Tris, 174
Tris-acetate, 209
Tris base, 207
Tris-Cl, 88, 104
Tris-HCl
  in direct sequencing by PCR, 155, 157, 158, 159
  in dot-blot differential hybridization, 115, 117
  in electrophoresis of DNA-protein complexes, 149
  in extraction of genomic DNA, 181, 182
  in isolation of plasmid DNA, 185, 186
  in preparation of insert DNA, 199
  in purification of mRNA, 193, 194
  in reporter gene analysis, 94, 95
Triton X-100, 95, 155
Trituration buffer, 204
Trypsin, 86
T7 primers, 53, 153, 196
T7 RNA polymerase sites, 50, 51, 115
T-tailed vectors, 110
T3 primers, 153, 196
Tube-to-tube variability, 44, 63, 77, 82, 90
Tubulin, 44, 82

U

Ultrapure Agarose, 208
Ultraviolet light, for decontamination, 8
Ultraviolet spectroscopy
  basic cloning by RT-PCR, 130
  in construction of PCR cloning vector, 54, 55
  in construction of TA cloning vector, 124
  ethidium bromide stain and, 207
  in extraction of genomic DNA, 181
  long-wavelength, 208
  in measurement of RNA, 195–196
United States Biochemical Corporation, 214

Upstream primer, definition, 44
Uracil deoxyribose N-glycosylase (UNG), 8
Urea, 188–189, 193

V

Vector pCRII, 110, 111, 112
Vent, 21, 29
Viruses, helper, 140

W

Wax-mediated hot start, 33, 34
Whatman DE81 filter, 78
Whatman 3MM filter, 106, 117, 149
Whitehead Institute, PRIMER software, 22, 26–28, 29
Wild-type plasmid, 55–57, 58, 59
Wizard Preps, 47, 50, 56, 58, 137
Worksheet templates, 74
World Wide Web sites. See Internet addresses
Worthington Biochemical Corporation, 214, 218
Wy-14,643-treated samples, 64

X

Xba1 restriction endonuclease site, 53, 127
X-Gal, 111, 126, 131, 158, 202, 203, 204
Xho1 restriction endonuclease site, 127
X-ray photography, 107, 110, 114, 149
Xylene, 87, 88
Xylene cyanol, 96, 106, 115, 159, 160, 209

Y

Yield, 28, 29, 30. See also Amplification efficiency
YT plus antibiotic, 112

Z

Zinc chloride, in preparation of insert DNA, 199